BORROWING LIFE

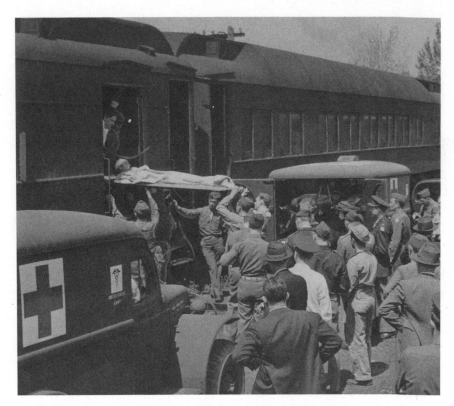

Wounded soldiers arriving by train at the Valley Forge Military Hospital
in Phoenixville, Pennsylvania, May, 1943

BORROWING LIFE

HOW SCIENTISTS, SURGEONS, AND A WAR HERO MADE
THE FIRST SUCCESSFUL ORGAN TRANSPLANT A REALITY

By Shelley Fraser Mickle

Photograph credits listed on page 271

An Imagine Book
Published by Charlesbridge
85 Main Street
Watertown, MA 02472
(617) 926-0329
www.imaginebooks.net

Cover and interior design by Ronaldo Alves

Library of Congress Cataloging-in-Publication Data
Names: Mickle, Shelley Fraser, author.
Title: Borrowing life : How scientists, surgeons, and a war hero made the first successful organ transplant a reality/ by Shelley Fraser Mickle.
Description: Watertown, MA : Charlesbridge, [2020] | Includes bibliographical references and index.
Identifiers: LCCN 2019015877 (print) | LCCN 2019019421 (ebook)
| ISBN 9781632892294 (ebook)
| ISBN 9781623545390 (reinforced for library use)
Subjects: LCSH: Kidneys—Transplantation—Boston—History. | Transplantation of organs, tissues, etc—History. | Peter Bent Brigham Hospital—History.
Classification: LCC RD575 (ebook) | LCC RD575 .M53 2020 (print) | DDC 617.4/610592—dc23
LC record available at https://lccn.loc.gov/2019015877

Printed in the United States of America
(hc) 10 9 8 7 6 5 4 3 2 1

For Parker

*Discovery consists of seeing what everybody has seen and
thinking what nobody has thought.*
—Albert Szent-Györgyi

Illness . . . has its inspirations.
—Albert Camus

Contents

PART III

A Note to Readers

THIS STORY BEGINS during World War II, six months after D-Day, when the worst fighting was still ahead. The Battle of the Bulge had just started; the crossing of the Rhine River was three months away. To tell it well, I must begin at an unexpected place. I say *unexpected* because when two young men came together that January of 1945—one a burned pilot, the other a surgeon determined to save him—they had no idea they were about to take the first step in making one of the most valuable contributions to mankind in the twentieth century.

While this story is mostly about what scientists and surgeons can achieve—given curiosity, a passion for science, a large dollop of compassion, and a little luck—it's a whole lot about how a science fiction-like dream pushed two American surgeons and a British scientist to scale the wall of what was deemed to be impossible. Over a decade they pioneered the giving and taking of organs that one of the surgeons called "spare-parts surgery," or borrowing life, which in no way belittled the ultimate gift of retrieving life for one so close to losing it.

In the late 1960s I knew two of the three. The American ones. I was too young and dumb to know I was walking among giants. The British one I know now by the energy of his words. And those of his wife, whose touching memoir gives us an idea of what it was like to love Peter Medawar, a scientist so important to the understanding of the universe of the immune system that his colleagues compared him to Galileo. Yes, Jean Medawar, like the wives of all these men, is unequivocally part of this narrative. As is Miriam Woods, who gives clear meaning to the words "in sickness and in health" as she devotedly rushed to be with her husband after a horrendous World War II plane crash. So here are four gripping love stories. In fact, before anyone answers that all-powerful question, *Will you marry me?*, they should ask: *Will you love me like Miriam loved Charles, like Joe loved Bobby, like Franny loved Laurie, like Jean loved Peter?*

Surgeon Joe Murray performed the first successful kidney transplant in December 1954 in a five-and-a-half-hour surgery—so monumental that it is immortalized in an oil painting hanging in the Countway Library in Boston next to the painting of the first surgery performed with ether. It is that important. Joe himself is a study in star stuff. At birth he was given gifts—those of both heredity and tradition. His family practiced irrepressible cheer as a matter of habit. His questing intelligence, unwavering buoyancy, uncommon dexterity, and an extraordinary compassion for those who suffered—especially for those who had to walk out into the world with a horrendous facial deformity, particularly children— seem almost superhuman. He said in his Nobel Prize lecture in 1990 that his life as a surgeon-scientist gave him the rewarding experience of witnessing "human nature in the raw: fear, despair, courage, understanding, hope, resignation, heroism." Indeed, his part in this story allows us to get our minds around the slippery concept of hope—and how not to lose it. Joe was not just one among many in the greatest generation, he was the kind of man who evokes prayers of *please God, make more like him.*

Francis ("Franny") Moore had the mettle of old New England running in his veins, the kind of grit that could make a man want to found a nation. Extraordinarily gifted as a surgeon-scientist, he was also extraordinarily gifted as a leader. And he had vision. He could foresee the promise of organ transplantation as a viable treatment for devastating injury and disease, thus opening the gates for the monumental first organ transplant in 1954. But that was not all. His understanding of how the body reacts to surgery still affects every patient who comes through a hospital door.

It was said that when Franny entered a room, it was like being in the midst of a full-scale orchestra performing a roof-raising symphony. He was that commanding. Paternal, wanting to take over and fix everything for everyone, he was loath to waste a minute, as if time and suffering were his enemies on the battlefield of sickness. Even his secretary said of him that "Dr. Moore lives life on a different plane." In short, he was like many esteemed people in history: he didn't have to do what he did. Born wealthy and privileged, he was driven by that elusive trait that we all wish for ourselves and for our children, and yet can't quite name. Simply put: *Get off your duff and pursue excellence for its own sake.* He would become the youngest surgeon to ever be named the Moseley Professor of Surgery at Harvard.

Peter Brian Medawar—how can we even grasp the whole of who he was? After witnessing a Spitfire crash near his home in Oxford, England, during the Battle of Britain, he became so haunted by the suffering of the burned pilot that he focused his brilliant mind on unveiling the secrets of the body's immune system to supply long-lasting skin grafts. His learning to bamboozle the body's system of defense to manipulate rejection established a new field of science, immunogenetics. In fact, Peter would make such a monumental contribution to the understanding of human biology that he was awarded the Nobel Prize in Medicine when he was only forty-five.

So here is this story: blending the horrors of war with the bold-ness of youth and the clenched-teeth defiance to not relinquish hope, it begins in December 1944 and will continue to be told well beyond today. Because borrowing life to extend the lives of those suffering from organ failure has enabled scientists of the present and future to apply the immune system's exquisite power to treating cancer and other ravaging diseases.

War—what is it good for? Beyond the absolute answer, *nothing*, there is that other little nudge: to find ways to preserve life. When historian Edward Gibbon wrote in the 1700s that "hope [is] the best comfort of our imperfect world," he knew what we humans were facing.

No, this is not quite a fairy tale, but it is close. The main differ-ence is that the villain is not human. It's death.

—Shelley Fraser Mickle
Spring, 2020

PART I

1

Joe

THE WOUNDED CAME EVERY DAY. They came straight from the front lines—from Europe, Africa, Italy, China, the Pacific. They came by trainloads in railroad cars, stacked in bunks, one over the other. Brought into the wards on gurneys, they soon swelled the Valley Forge Military Hospital in Phoenixville, Pennsylvania, into the largest in the United States: three thousand patients. A hundred buildings. Tunnels connected the buildings to outfox the weather. Day and night, the staff never stopped moving.

That fall of 1944, a young man briskly walked through the halls. Like all medical students in America, he had been drafted after Japan's attack on Pearl Harbor. Slim, athletic, a few inches under six feet, Joe Murray was swallowed up by the official uniform of all medical personnel. At a distance, you might even mistake his heavily starched white coat and pants to be walking on their own.

At twenty-five, after only nine months of surgical training, he had been assigned to Valley Forge to await overseas duty. When first called up, he'd tried to join the navy. But because of his myopia, he was turned away, and the army became his only option. He was still laughing at the irony that for all his childhood photographs, his mother had dressed him in sailor suits.

With his rimless glasses reflecting the glare of the overhead hospital lights, he did not seem anything other than the prized student of his fifth-grade class in Milford, Massachusetts, or the salutatorian at his high school graduation. He was simply too understated to catch much attention. His presence was akin to the subtle movement of the earth's seasons. He was that constant, that reliable, that fueled by a hidden power. Over the more than ninety years that he would live, he would keep many of the traits he showed as a callow young lieutenant at the beginning of the war—humming songs as he worked, upbeat, quick to connect with others by asking, "And where are you from?" Of course, the songs would change, and in the 1960s he would begin singing his favorite Louis Armstrong song, "What a Wonderful World," his tenor voice delivering words that expressed exactly his view on life: "I hear babies cry, I watch them grow . . . and I think to myself what a wonderful world." Eventually he would have six children over seventeen years, so those words would take on richer meaning. And after his first grandchildren discovered his gentle nature and grand achievements, they poked fun at him by nicknaming him "Holy Joe."

Yes, throughout the years of his long life, he would stay much as he was that winter of 1944: wiry, thin, athletic, and fearless. His questing intelligence could be daunting. As his brown hair disappeared, friends would say that his head was simply too occupied to grow hair—grass doesn't grow on a busy street! His reverence for all life never waned. He would continue to pry an insect from a window screen and flick it outside rather than squash it. To eat burned toast for breakfast. To drink chocolate syrup straight from the can. And to give no reasons. The delight in such childlike whimsy was its own excuse for being.

Indeed, he was so unassuming and cheerful, few would guess that he was fueled by a secret sweet stubbornness. Not the bullheaded sort that could stop action, but the unrelenting kind that could calmly spend hours picking a rusty lock to release whatever was captive. From his Irish grandparents and Italian mother he learned a cheerfulness that perhaps only immigrants fully understand. To them, getting into America was a lucky charm that pessimism should never tarnish, so Joe grew up in a household with the Pollyannaish outlook that every glass was not just half full but a fountain, overflowing. Already, in his twenties, he had a spray of smile lines at the edges of his glasses and parentheses of smile tracks around his mouth.

That winter of 1944, as he went from room to room at the Valley Forge Hospital checking on patients, he probably hummed tunes from that year's hit parade, "Sentimental Journey" and "Don't Fence Me In." Music was his passion—as well as a lingering desire. While in medical school, he had walked to the Boston Conservatory to take piano lessons until his unrelenting honesty demanded that he quit. Explaining away his small talent with characteristic humor, he said he was going to marry musical talent instead. Indeed, his fiancée, Bobby Link, was studying piano and voice. The following June they were to be married in a church in upstate New York, and Joe's greatest worry was being sent overseas. Being separated from Bobby would be agony.

Thankfully, work at Valley Forge kept his mind distracted from *that*. The sheer number of patients was daunting. With only nine months of surgical training, he was barely prepared for a normal hospital, much less one like this. Five days a week, from eight in the morning to three in the afternoon, three operating rooms were running with two surgeries performed in each. By the end of the day, Joe often had completed twenty to twenty-five operations. After each, the used instruments were taken away, sterilized, and quickly brought back, so that in five to ten minutes he could begin the next.

And the wounded never stopped coming.

Since outstanding surgeons were brought to Valley Forge from across the country, the military hospital provided a great education. By a quirk of nature, Joe was garnering notice in the operating room, for he was left-handed, and since his elementary school teachers had insisted he conform to a right-handed world, he was now ambidextrous. He could conquer puzzles of anatomy by getting into tight spots in ways that other surgeons couldn't. He could use both right- and left-handed surgical instruments, which meant he never had to change his angle of attack. To get at a patient from the other side, he didn't have to walk around the operating table, which saved that patient from more time under anesthesia.

Most of all, his thoughts centered on Bobby. Starting off their married life in this countryside of rolling hills, surrounded by Amish and Mennonite communities, would be idyllic. Because of gas rationing, he carpooled the twenty miles from his rented cottage to the hospital with a technician who also worked there, and they often passed horse-drawn buggies. Hardships of war would not be hardships but problems to solve.

Housekeeping would be a puzzle. Tires, gasoline, meat, butter, canned vegetables, sugar, shoes—all were rationed. Ration cards had been issued to over a hundred million Americans. Corn syrup was a substitute for sugar. Most civilians grew their own vegetables in victory gardens because food was needed for the troops. By 1943, there were some twenty million victory gardens throughout the United States. But Joe and Bobby had already agreed to brush wartime difficulties aside. They felt optimistic and hoped for a large family.

He could hardly wait to have Bobby in Phoenixville with him.

The previous June, after the invasion of Normandy, the Allied forces were aiming for the Rhine River, hoping to cross it in March. The Battle of the Bulge had started in December 1944. The year before, when General Eisenhower announced the surrender of Italy on September 8, 1943, Hitler had sent his troops swarming into the Italian countryside because the Allies were so close to the German-occupied Balkans. The fighting there turned especially vicious. In the winter of 1943–44, US soldiers faced agonies that few Americans knew about.

GIs battled not just German troops but also frostbite. Trench foot was epidemic. The war was now a war of attrition. Dead bodies were wrapped in bloody bed sacks, waiting for pickup. Scavenging dogs ate the throats of the dead, while at home in America, people were noting how the war had lifted the grip of the Great Depression. War production sent money flowing.

As a first lieutenant at Valley Forge, Joe had no control over his future. He had no idea where he would be sent. What he knew above all else was that having to leave Bobby to go overseas would be the most pain he could ever experience.

What he did not know was that, during that first winter in Valley Forge, he would meet a young pilot, who, as they worked together to cheat death, would change both their lives and lay the groundwork for borrowing life in the give-and-take of human organs.

To achieve that, he would need someone to balance out his gentle nature. He needed a protector, some bold fellow-surgeon to step forward, one who was willing to buck traditional thinking, to clear the way.

2

Charles

AT ONLY TWENTY-TWO, Charles Woods was a crackerjack pilot, so good that he was instructing other pilots, not just in flying, but in "Flying the Hump"—one of the most necessary and dangerous missions in World War II.

He was tall, just under six feet, and handsome. Resembling the soldier Audie Murphy, the war hero turned movie star, Charles would become known *not* for the medals he acquired, but for what he had lost.

The morning of December 23, 1944, he was asleep on a cot in a tent at the airbase in Kurmitola, India. It was four o'clock in the morning. Five hours before, he had returned from a round trip to Lyuliang, China, where he had delivered 28,000 gallons of aviation fuel to the US pilots known as the Flying Tigers. Too tired to change clothes, he had simply fallen asleep in his flight suit, and now he felt a hand shaking him awake to fly the route again.

Never before had there been anything like this long-range, around-the-clock mission. When Nazi Germany invaded Poland in September 1939, marking the official beginning of World War II, China had already been at war with Japan for two years. In a covert mission directed by President Franklin Roosevelt, nonmilitary pilots were hired to fly combat missions against the Japanese. These were known as the Flying Tigers, hunkering down in China, unknown to the public, secret and fierce. After the Japanese attack on Pearl Harbor prompted America to enter the war, the Flying Tigers officially became part of the US military. Above board, heroic now, helping China drive out the Japanese, they would eventually inspire a movie, starring John Wayne.

Since there was no airfield in the China–Burma area from which to deliver fuel to the Tigers in Lyuliang, US pilots flew the lifeblood fuel from Kurmitola. The route was five hundred miles over the Himalayan Mountains, hence the name, "Flying the Hump." It was as challenging as flying ever gets, which was why Charles wanted to fly it. Dream-bitten with the idea of being a pilot since a young boy, he was now considered among the best.

Flying the Hump was a hazardous route. There were no radio navigation aids, and the weather was always abysmal. If it wasn't snowing in the Himalayas, it was sleeting. There were surging updrafts and wind shears. To avoid ice forming on his plane's wings and frosting his windshield, Charles figured out that he could drop his plane into the lower mountain peaks where the air was warmer. He flew the Hump every day. Already he had flown it more than a hundred times, and he never dwelled on the dangers. The planes were B-24 Liberators converted from bombers to fuel carriers. With four engines and three-bladed propellers, the planes had huge gas containers snuggled in their bellies. The delivery of each plane's 28,000 gallons of fuel was a lifeline for the Tigers, a significant hope for the Chinese suffering brutal Japanese aerial attacks. Cit ies were bombed, killing hundreds. Chinese citizens stacked up the bodies of their dead like cordwood to line the streets. The Flying Tigers were a critical line of defense for the Chinese, defending them from Japanese attacks, and Charles was a link in that lifeline.

Now he was teaching other pilots his tricks, sharpening their skills to Fly the Hump. And stay alive.

Planes were frequently lost in the peaks of the Himalayas. The statistics for all combat pilots told the cold reality: fighter and bomber pilots in Europe were so often lost that their average combat life expectancy was fifty-six flying hours. With every mission, more than 10 percent of the planes were lost. Each pilot averaged two missions a week, so that the life expectancy of a World War II pilot was only thirty days. For those Flying the Hump, the statistics were even worse. Every ninety days, 100 percent of the planes were lost. For this reason, pilots did not expect to live long, and they kept to themselves. Rarely making friends was a given. Hanging out at the officers' club was not their habit, either. They were too tired. They ate, slept, and flew. Of the danger, Charles said, "I tried not to think about it. I accepted it as part of my job, and when I was told to fly, I flew."

With those harsh statistics, the army was constantly in need of pilots. So, Charles's job as an instructor was to make sure there was a steady supply for the mission. Not just the route, but the combat flying hours were also brutal: 140 to 150 combat hours every month. Compared to today's commercial pilots, who are restricted to resting after flying 100 hours, Charles was piling up unheard of records. Often, while the Chinese drained the fuel from the planes into their holding tanks, the Hump pilots would lie down under the wing of their plane and take a nap, then remount the cockpit to start back to hand off the next five-hundred-mile trip to another American pilot.

Maybe Charles's grim childhood gave him the grit to take on such a mission. When his divorced mother struggled to support him and his older brother, she placed the boys in an orphanage near their home in Alabama. Charles was five, and he never saw his mother again. A year later, when a loving family adopted him, he lost touch with his brother, too. The scar of being abandoned never completely faded. No wonder a dream of leaving his troubles— soaring above earth in silent air except for the comforting roar of engines that could keep him airborne—took hold of him, and took hold of him hard.

Right after graduating from high school, he took a bus to Windsor, Ontario, to enlist in the Royal Canadian Air Force. In 1940, Canada, as part of the British Commonwealth, was already at war with Germany. The Canadian military was eager for young men, and Charles was eager for the chance to learn to fly.

For him, basic training in Canada was a snap. He had abundant talent to fuel his pilot dreams. After graduation, skilled and ready as a Canadian Air Force pilot, armed with the invincibility of being barely twenty, he spent the next two years flying missions in England and North Africa.

Nearly a year before America entered the war, an impromptu meeting caught him off guard. Totally unexpected and deeply affecting, the experience knocked him into unknown territory that can be summed up by one word: Miriam.

January 3, 1941, eight o'clock in the evening. Nearly a year before the Japanese attack on Pearl Harbor, Charles was visiting his home in Alabama from the Canadian Air Force base, when a friend set him up on a blind date. She was small, eighteen years old.

"Where you from?" he asked her.

"Hartford," she said.

"That's just around the corner from where I live! How come I haven't seen you around?"

"Maybe you weren't looking."

Her playfulness and sass were exactly the traits that made Charles know this girl named Miriam was very likely his match.

After all, when he had been living at the orphanage, his spirited daring became legend. One day he stuck a safety pin in the lock to the door that led to the orphanage roof. When it opened, he directed other kids up behind him just to see what they could see. Even after he was caught and punished, he never regretted taking the risk.

For two years, he dated Miriam. After America entered the war, when he switched to the Army Air Corps and was assigned to India to Fly the Hump, he married her. They had a son, and it was this family and Miriam's daily letters that brightened his days at the airbase in Kurmitola. Since Irving Berlin's song "White Christmas" had come out in 1942, it was playing in a lot of places that December, expressing soldiers' longing to be home, and the song had become a beloved wartime standard.

Two days before Christmas, the song was being heard almost everywhere, and Charles assumed he would be spending the holiday in India, alone.

On that morning of December 23, 1944, a jeep took him and his crew out to his plane. It was not yet daylight. The runway was lit, bordered with lights. Since he had already served two years with the Canadian Air Force, flying in Europe and North Africa, he didn't really need to sign up with the US Army Air Corps after the Pearl Harbor attack. But he had his reasons, and they all had to do with what he foresaw Hitler doing.

To him, Hitler was more than a funny little man with a mustache. He feared what Hitler's victories could mean, that the dictator's designs on world domination threatened America. He agreed with what President Roosevelt made clear in his speeches: that air power made an invasion of America possible, that all democracies were in peril. Charles saw the dangers to the world through the same lens as the president, and re-enlisted. Being assigned to

Fly the Hump was an honor; it meant he was one of the best. His recent assignment to teach new pilots what he already knew about the mission increased the risks. But turning the controls over to an inexperienced pilot-in-training was part of his job.

That morning, the new pilot was a young captain named Stalmacher.

For a dozen flights, Stalmacher had never been commander of a mission over the Himalayas. He had always been a copilot. This was his day to earn a plane of his own.

No doubt he shared the same love of risk and daring as all pilots. A hunger for being on the edge—when you don't really ever believe, not really, that you will lose your life—made up the moments that infused living with a deep realization of being alive. This was the characteristic all pilots shared. And Charles had that characteristic in abundance. Stalmacher, too, except perhaps he also was inclined to overthink things and prepare too methodically. A pilot, similar to a surgeon, cannot be timid. Acting boldly, buoyed by superhuman confidence, surgeons and pilots share traits of daring and love of danger. The good ones have a propensity for ignoring all other reality but the job at hand—and succeeding.

Stalmacher was chatting about how he thought he'd soon be given his own plane. In the back of the jeep were Donald Hoag, the flight engineer, and Skip Rodriguez, the radio operator.

The four men climbed into the plane: Hoag and Rodriguez in the rear and Woods and Stalmacher in the cockpit. It was still dark, and the lighted six-thousand-foot asphalt runway was like a ribbon cutting through the Indian jungle.

Charles said his usual takeoff prayer: *Dear God, please be with us,* and then removed his gloves and helmet, as most aviators did, to give him more dexterity and closer vision on takeoff. The fact that he did would have disastrous consequences in a matter of minutes.

Stalmacher revved the engine. The propellers began loudly turning.

The plane's takeoff power increased, and Stalmacher moved the plane to the head of the runway. Charles called off the two-page checklist, talking to Hoag and Rodriguez on the intercom. He radioed the tower: "B-24 ready for takeoff."

"Have a good flight," the controller said, his usual reply. The takeoff ritual seemed to diminish the mission's life-or-death danger.

Stalmacher punched the throttle while holding the brakes as the engines reached full power. With 28,000 gallons of fuel weighing 65,000 pounds, the plane needed plenty of runway to take off. It was like a lumbering elephant. To become airborne, the B-24 would have to reach 120 miles an hour.

Charles reminded Stalmacher of this. "Don't worry about me, captain," Stalmacher replied, smiling. "I can handle her all right."

"I figured you could," Charles encouraged.

The plane sped down the runway. Stalmacher, despite his attempts to seem relaxed, wasn't. He came off as too careful, robotically following a script and not operating on intuition and feel. For a moment Charles thought that, as commander, he could pull the flight and go back. But what would be his excuse: that Stalmacher wasn't ready? After all, Stalmacher was a pilot-in-training. It was Charles's job to see that these pilots-in-training reached the next level.

Still, Charles was concerned; he had a feeling, a gut feeling, a foreboding. But he overrode it.

Seeing the dial register a hundred miles per hour, Stalmacher lifted the plane's nose. "She's too high," called out Charles.

Stalmacher lowered the nose.

"One hundred ten," said Charles. "One hundred fifteen. One hundred twenty."

As Charles yelled "One hundred twenty," Stalmacher pushed the brakes with his feet, thinking the plane was in the air and that he needed to stop the wheels from spinning. Suddenly, the nose of the plane pitched forward.

In that moment, the speed dropped to ninety miles an hour. There was less than six hundred feet of runway left. Not enough to build up again to the 120-mile-an-hour takeoff speed.

Charles reached for the controls. He had three choices. He could slam down on one brake, making the aircraft spin around. The gear would break loose. The gas tanks would probably rupture, and the plane would explode. Or, he could pull back on the control wheel and gamble on lifting the craft off the ground. But whenever that maneuver had been used with a B-24, the plane had stalled and rolled into a ball of fire.

In those crashes, no one survived.

Charles decided his best chance was to shut off the power, stand on the brakes to reduce the plane's speed so that when it rolled off the runway, it would sink into the dirt. If the plane were moving slowly enough, and if Charles could keep it on a straight path, it might come to rest without ripping a fuel tank.

He yanked off the power and stood on the brakes. He fought the controls as the plane plowed off the runway into the dirt at the end, scraping off the nose wheels and gear.

Stalmacher was battling the controls on his side of the cabin, too. The plane skidded ahead, straight, scraping a wide swath in the Indian jungle next to the runway. It slowed to sixty miles an hour, fifty, forty, thirty-five, thirty. It was coming to a stop. But then the plane shuddered as it hit a fallen tree. Gasoline spewed out. A spark set it off. Charles yelled to the crew, "Let's get out of here!"

The fuel tank exploded, and a hurricane of flames swept over them.

Charles held his breath and closed his eyes, hoping to spare them from the flames. He began unfastening his seat belt. He opened his eyes briefly and saw Stalmacher beating at flames on his flight suit.

With his eyes shut again, Charles slid the panel on the cockpit open and lunged forward to let his weight carry him ten feet below to the burning ground.

Breaking his fall with his hands, he rolled over and sprang to his feet. He ran for the darkness beyond the circle of fire. He turned to look back at the plane. Only the tips of the wings were visible. The rest of the big B-24 lay disintegrating inside the inferno.

Acting on reflex, thinking there was nothing else to do, he sat on a mound of dirt to wait for his crewmates. Seeing the cuffs and neck of his flight suit smoldering, he slapped out the fire with his hands.

Soon people from small houses and shacks on the outskirts of the field surrounded him. Several helped him pull off his flight suit. Two others removed his paratrooper boots. His eyes swelled shut. "Does anybody speak English?" he asked.

"Yes," a voice said. "I'm British."

"Could you see about getting me an ambulance?" As soon as he said it, he regretted it. What did he need an ambulance for?

"Straight away, sir," someone said.

Then he added, "Has anybody seen the other men in my crew?" Nobody answered.

He was the only one who made it out. And only later would he realize how severely he was burned.

3

Franny

TWO YEARS BEFORE, on the Saturday after Thanksgiving, radio stations were broadcasting football championships all across America. Francis Moore, twenty-nine years old, affectionately nicknamed Franny, was on call as a surgical resident at Massachusetts General Hospital in downtown Boston.

The night had been slow with few demands on his time. He was in the upstairs residents' lounge listening to the games. Unlike Joe, he had been exempt from the military draft because of bronchial asthma he'd battled since childhood. Told that "your job is right here," essential to the home front, he'd gone straight from medical school into his internship and residency. And now, after graduating from Harvard Medical School in 1939, he was on his way to being a surgeon.

With America at war, surgical training was compressed from the usual five or six years to twenty-seven months, a severe challenge. Teaching hospitals were turning out surgeons for the war effort by the thousands. Harvard Medical School would not admit a woman until 1945, but nurses were in great need and their training was expedited as well, most often to four weeks.

Tall, with dark hair to eventually turn a distinguishing silver, Franny came from men and women who settled in Vermont, Maine, and Boston—all well-educated, successful, and resourceful. While his father and grandfathers were hard-driving and high-achieving, it was his mother, Caroline Seymour Daniels, who was the intellectual in the family. Educated in Connecticut and Vermont, she read the classics in both Latin and Greek and was always ready to engage in a lively intellectual discussion on any topic. Along with these inherited traits of intellect and temperament, Franny also had an imposing physical presence. His handsome, patrician features—longish nose, oval face, intense but kind eyes—were coupled with a resonant voice. His take-charge air became, in short, that old slippery thing we call charisma. To him life was music, well done, a performance to echo. In a sense, he embodied the traditional New England virtues of ambition, humility, and a dry wit.

With not a jot of athletic ability whatsoever, he had long, dexterous fingers that, paired with a musical talent, could fly over a piano keyboard. He was even adept enough as a musician to write a musical for the Hasty Pudding Club when he was an undergraduate at Harvard. He played the piano to accompany the cast singers and in April 1934 took the show on the road.

While the cast performed his musical, *Hades! The Ladies?*, he sat at the piano, playing cheerfully, nodding along, his eyes connecting with the singers to keep them in rhythm. When Eleanor Roosevelt heard that the show was on the road, she invited them to the White House for tea in the East Room. Franny played the piano while the cast sang. And since he'd looked up the Hasty Pudding show in which Franklin Roosevelt, as an undergraduate at Harvard, had played the part of a chorus girl, Franny and the cast sang some of the president's songs. The president's famous bellowing laugh, no doubt, roared through the White House.

As the son of one of America's ingenious entrepreneurs, Franny didn't have to worry that as a surgical resident he was making only twenty-five dollars a month with a wife and young children to support. Even he would admit that he had grown up spoiled: household help, chauffeurs, summer vacations in New England and Wyoming, fine cars, the best education. In the early 1900s, his father had drifted from New England to Chicago where he bought a patent for a rail anchor, known as an anticreeper, to keep a rail from rippling under the wheels of a heavy train. From that, his family became not just financially secure, but wealthy, eventually buying a large house in an affluent area outside of Chicago on the shore of Lake Michigan.

At twelve, Franny had appendicitis. At fourteen, he had a busted knee. Admiring the surgeon who took care of him, he saw that few could claim such an exemplary life. He saw competence, the ability to relieve pain, and the reverence given to men of medicine. His eventual decision to become a surgeon was not grounded in ambitions that his parents had for him. He simply saw surgery as the most fascinating and rapidly advancing field of science. But he was also caught by something more difficult to describe, something that mellowed his take-charge temperament. It modulated his natural showmanship, filled him with a bottomless supply of compassion, and propelled him toward excellence—at least in her eyes: Laurie.

As if thrown off a cliff, the shock of falling in love was a force he could not control. At fifteen, he was mired in a mix of lust, the certainty of a soul mate for life, and an irreversible need to have her—not just temporarily but forever. A year younger, petite Laurie was an only child of wealthy parents. Her elfin face, short brown, wavy hair, and steady eyes spoke of a steadfast character and a ready playfulness, which Franny knew attracted not just him. Everyone fell in love with her, so he had to hurry to snap her up. Since she lived in a large house about a mile from his parents' home, he would borrow the family car to drive there almost every night, all through high school. After a couple of years, his father said that when anyone else got behind the wheel of the car, it would automatically go to Laurie's.

The intensity of their relationship lasted through Franny's four years at Harvard and Laurie's college years at Sarah Lawrence, remaining so strong that just before he began his first year of medical school, they announced they wanted to get married. No one was surprised. Marrying so early in a medical career was almost unheard of. Franny didn't care. And his and Laurie's parents made it financially possible.

On that night of November 28, 1942, when Laurie was home, looking after their young family, Franny was at Massachusetts General Hospital with the football radio broadcast winding down. At ten-thirty he heard the whine of a siren. Hearing a siren heading to Mass General was not uncommon. But then, he heard the whine of another, then another and another.

Quickly, he put on his white coat and ran downstairs, holding his pocket to keep his stethoscope from falling out. By the time he walked into the hall leading to the emergency room, dead bodies were lined up in rows. The smell of burned clothes and hair permeated that side of the building.

Only three years out of medical school, he was swept up in a tragedy of historic proportions. Indeed, the Cocoanut Grove fire would be one of the worst civilian disasters in American history. Going from patient to patient, overwhelmed with so many to help, he saw nurses trying to relieve the overwhelming pain of those with burns. They gave morphine freely, sometimes overdosing victims and hastening their deaths. Other nurses began writing an *M* in lipstick on the foreheads of patients to prevent duplicate doses of morphine.

Several hours later Franny finally learned exactly what had happened. A thousand young people had crowded into the Cocoanut Grove nightclub, most of them soldiers with their sweethearts, to celebrate the holiday break before going overseas. And to rib each other over the football scores in the title games.

The nightclub, near the center of downtown Boston, close to Boston Common, was under new management. Redecorated with imitation palm trees and drapes, it was overcrowded that night. At about ten-fifteen some of the decorations caught fire, and within five minutes the entire nightclub was an inferno. More than four hundred people died instantly. The fire, much like the fuel explosion from Charles's crash, spread through the nightclub within seconds, stoked by the flammable drapes. It likely started in a basement lounge, possibly from a match or a cigarette. The burning decorations and drapes set off chemical reactions. Instantly, oxygen was used up in the tightly closed restaurant and carbon monoxide filled the building. Carbon monoxide poisoning turns human blood cherry pink rather than deep red. The faces of some of those who reached the hospital only minutes from dying had that deceptively healthy-looking color.

Burning wall paint and dyes in the drapes set off poisonous gases, leading to effects similar to those World War I soldiers suffered from mustard-gas poisoning. One naval officer, who made it to the hospital from the fire, ran from room to room looking for his friends and collapsed, dying from the secretions in his lungs that drowned him.

The fire department put out the flames within thirty minutes, but the tragedy was so awful that radio newscasts kept repeating the details. The public was horrified. Of the four hundred who died, a large number succumbed to suffocation so suddenly that they were found sitting at tables, unburned, rigid in death, clutching drink glasses.

Two months after the fire, Franny was still treating nine severely burned patients in the hospital. Eventually one of the nightclub owners was judged guilty of negligence and sent to prison.

While learning how to treat fluid loss, burn shock, infection, and respiratory tract injury, how to perform grafting, and how to monitor a dozen body chemicals, Franny became an expert in burn therapy. For the next five years, the navy and army funded his research with the side effect that his heroic role in the tragedy, and his guidance in preparing for other disasters, made him nationally known. And revered.

Two years later, his advancements in treating burns were known to other physicians, especially to those at the burn unit at Valley Forge. And Joe, equipped with that knowledge, was following the latest protocol for the young men who came every day, straight from the battlefields, horribly burned. Most were pilots. Most were hanging onto life by sheer will, like Charles.

This first contribution of knowledge that Franny passed on to Joe would be the lead-in to a career that would connect Charles, Franny, Joe, and a young scientist in Britain who also saw horrors of war he could never forget.

4

Death Was Unacceptable

WHEN JOE WALKED into the room at the Valley Forge Hospital where Charles lay, he saw a pilot, three years younger than he was, with no nose, no eyelids, no ears, and only a raw opening where his mouth had been. This was the worst burn case Joe had ever seen. Ordinarily, someone burned this severely would not live but a few moments after the fire.

But there was Charles, burned over most of his body, his face completely erased by the fire, and teetering on the edge of life. Clearly, he was holding on with teeth-clenched defiance. Recognizing this, Joe immediately knew that losing Charles was not acceptable. Not only was he young and deserving of life and quality of life, but he had already fought so hard to stay alive.

As the youngest of four physicians to take care of Charles, Joe acquired most of his knowledge about the treatment for burns from articles Franny had published in academic journals. Those studies informed the Valley Forge burn unit, so they all knew the most immediate danger to Charles was suffocation. The swelling in his burned airway was restricting air flow. Right away they placed tubes in his lungs to keep the air coming, and then they turned their attention to the fluids leaking from his burn wounds.

Skin is the body's ultimate protection—holding in fluids and keeping out foreign invaders—and Charles had little dermal layer left to shield him. He was burned over 70 percent of his body.

His body's fluids were leaking out. He was dying of dehydration. The only way to stop the loss and build a protection against infection was to quickly take healthy skin from some part of his body to graft over his wounds. Known as *autografts*, those self-harvested skin bandages were standard treatment for burns. But Charles was burned so severely, he had no healthy skin available to harvest. Furthermore, he was too weak to withstand such an operation. A single alternative was left: borrowing skin from someone else. Taking skin from another body and surgically applying it in what is known as an *allograft* was only a stopgap measure. It was well known that in ten to fourteen days, that skin would shrink, turn gray, and slough off in the process of rejection when the body perceived the borrowed skin to be foreign. However, there was always the chance that an allograft could buy enough time for scar to form to stave off fluid loss and infection, and hence save a life. The process had been witnessed for centuries. *Why* tissue rejection happened no one knew. *How* was even more of a mystery. But centuries of medical history had documented the short life of allografts, and there were no exceptions.

Only in one situation had borrowed skin been found to escape rejection and that was skin shared between identical twins. Eight years before, Dr. James Barrett Brown, a plastic surgeon in St. Louis, had cross-grafted skin of identical twins, establishing that allografts could be traded back and forth between them with perfect success.

But Charles had no twin.

As he lay close to death that January of 1945, he was running a constant fever. Knowledge from Franny's research forewarned that burn victims who made it through the first threat of suffocation were, almost always, killed by infection. At the time of the nightclub fire, penicillin was an experimental drug. But with the advent of World War II, it had become essential.

A serendipitous 1928 discovery that mold released a substance that repressed bacteria led to the discovery of penicillin, but the miracle drug was not available to the general public. In June 1942, there was only enough penicillin to treat ten patients from the Cocoanut Grove fire. However, by July 1943, the War Production Board had drawn up a plan to use new research of fermentation on corn steep liquor to mass-produce the miracle antibiotic. In a worldwide search for a mold to kick-start mass production, a moldy cantaloupe was found in a market in Peoria, Illinois. That melon, along with the new-found fermentation method, allowed 2.3 million doses of penicillin to be produced in time for the invasion of Normandy in June 1944—also just in time for Charles to benefit the following December.

On his trip to the States, he had been given several doses. As Joe studied the young pilot with his devastating injuries, he realized that Charles had used up all his strength getting back to the States, and infection threatened to sap the rest. The trip from India to Valley Forge had been brutal.

Right after the crash, Charles had been lifted onto a cargo plane and flown two hundred miles away to a hospital in Calcutta. His record as a courageous pilot gave him priority status to be rushed to the Valley Forge Hospital, the best for the treatment of burns. But that was ten thousand miles away.

Charles was so weak that he could fly only one day. He would then have to rest in a hospital somewhere. With no eyelids, he could not blink to keep his eyes moist. Nurses were constantly applying Vaseline to his eyes, then bandaging them. Gauze and tape covered his face and hands. He could rely only on the sound of voices around him to know what was happening.

At each stop, a forklift removed his stretcher on a wooden platform, and he was taken into an infirmary for a small meal of baby food and to have his bandages replaced. Several times he heard people talking around him as if he were already dead.

The cargo planes were bumpy and torturous. He was jiggled and bumped. For a while, there was no pain. He figured his nerve endings must have been seared in the fire, and he was numb. But after a few weeks, the pain started. At first, he asked for painkillers, and then feared becoming addicted and willed himself to withstand the pain by traveling in his mind from one memory to another.

From Calcutta, he was flown to rest in Basra, Iraq, and then to Cairo and Casablanca. Finally, for the last leg of the journey, he was assigned a full-time nurse who helped keep him hydrated. The pilot of the plane also climbed to a higher altitude to make a smoother ride for him. Stopping to refuel in Reykjavik, the cargo plane then sped toward the hospital in Pennsylvania. The trip had taken six agonizing weeks.

Now Joe and the team of doctors knew they had to think outside the box to build Charles a dermal layer. And to do so immediately. They needed to find a donor. Even though in a matter of a week Charles's body could perceive the transplanted skin as foreign, and his immune system would attack and kill it, an allograft was worth risking to save his life.

As the team of four was considering what to do, one suggested they might take skin from a cadaver. Even with so many sick men in the Valley Forge Hospital, the likelihood that a dying man could become Charles's donor in time to save him seemed a long shot. But it was the only one they had.

5

Peter

IN SEPTEMBER 1939, Peter Medawar, a twenty-four-year-old zoology graduate student, was living in a rented house in Oxford, England, with his wife, Jean, and their young daughter. They were all on the back lawn, Peter reading, Jean working in the vegetable garden, when they heard a plane and looked up to see it coming over the rooftops toward them. Jean picked up their daughter, and they all rushed into the homemade bomb shelter in the basement.

War with Germany had just been declared. Oxford was swamped with London evacuees. German planes had been bombing London but were rarely expected in Oxford. Still, it was a horrifying sight to see the plane coming toward them and to think it might be German, stocked with bombs.

The British service had not called up Peter. The recruiting board had said that as a scientist he should undertake research that might be "of service to the medical establishment"—meaning anything that could treat war wounds. Peter himself suspected that the real reason was that his feet were too big to fit into the military boots issued to inductees. His feet matched his six-foot-five height and, as he liked to say with self-deprecating wit, were also "flat," which probably would have disqualified him from combat anyway.

Like everyone else, when the war was declared, he and Jean hunkered down—draping their house windows with blackout curtains and practicing food rationing, even raising their own supply of chickens. But when they found themselves too tender-hearted to wring their chicken's necks, they comically used leftover ether from Peter's lab.

Stoically, they had even prepared themselves for the worst. When Hitler's Minister for Propaganda, Joseph Goebbels, began making radio broadcasts laying out his ideas on racial purity, Peter surmised that if Germany won the recent air attacks on Britain, he would qualify for the Nazi firing squad. His father was Lebanese; his complexion was dark.

That day, after Peter heard the roar of a bomber and shepherded his young family into their homemade air-raid shelter, he waited, staying calm for the sake of Jean and their daughter, while listening for what was happening outside. Soon, they heard a loud thump and a horrifying explosion.

Running out, Peter saw the plane had crashed in their neighbor's garden. The flames were rooftop high, rising over the neighborhood. It was British, flown by one of the Spitfire pilots defending against Hitler's Luftwaffe.

The neighbors pulled the young airman out and rushed him to the nearby hospital. Sixty percent of his body was burned. With his physicians at their wits' end for what they could do for him, one suggested to Peter that "he lay aside his intellectual pursuits and take a serious interest in real life." He asked Peter to think about the burned pilot and come up with some bright ideas as to how he might be treated.

Peter returned to the hospital to visit the young pilot and saw things he could not un-see. Wavering on the edge of life, the man's suffering was haunting. Shaken, Peter realized his scientific background was a means to develop new treatments. He knew that skin grafts were the only way to outlast dehydration and infection. So, why not make skin grafts last longer? Why not prevent rejection? Why not find a way to successfully borrow skin from an unrelated donor? Why not pursue the underlying questions to find answers that would be far-reaching and elemental? Why not probe the mysteries to ask and answer *how* exactly does the body tell the difference between its own and other living cells? How does the body discriminate between *self* and *non-self*?

His mind had always been so restless. So fidgety with its constant need to make sense of things! Here now was a place for his questing intellect to land, to take hold of a subject that could benefit untold millions, as well as to last far beyond his own lifespan. He now asked himself, "How could I allow myself to fritter away my time as I did?"

It was then he decided that he would have no more of those experiments he called "messings about." From that moment, his career as a scientist was fixed.

Armed with a pair of dissecting scissors, a few rabbits, and mice, Peter practically began living in a dilapidated laboratory. Since he knew the process of rejection was too complicated to unravel in time to help the young pilot, his first focus was on multiplying usable skin over the burned pilot's own body.

Obsessed with unlocking biology's secrets, he stayed at the lab until late at night, joking that he kept the night watchmen and cleaning staff from being lonely. His unique scientific strength came from his student days when he had spent long hours learning the technique of tissue culture. Growing living cells outside the body at body temperature and in a nutrient culture medium had been going on for a decade, but using tissue culture to solve biological problems had not gotten off the ground. Thus far, scientists had been delighted and beguiled by the sheer beauty of the cultivated cells under a microscope.

As a student, Peter had spent long hours doing bench science—work in the laboratory with no patient contact—learning to preserve and harden tissues for microscopic study. Realizing that he had to master the orthodox technique for culturing tissues, he dehydrated and impregnated them with paraffin wax and used a precision instrument to cut them into slices of a thousandth of a millimeter thick. Then he mounted the very thin slices on glass slides and stained them with a variety of natural or synthetic dyes to bring out the various structures in the tissues that differentiated them. He became so adept at this bench science that when one of his revered professors remarked one day that he was writing a history of the use of dyes in preparing tissues for microscopic observation, Peter, still a graduate student, offhandedly offered, "I expect you [know] Leeuwenhoek used saffron as a microscopic stain." His professor was stunned by the breadth of Peter's knowledge, even of the obscure methods used by the Dutch pioneer who developed the microscope. It was clear that Peter was a step ahead, already in a realm that few scientists could match.

But mainly there had never been anyone before who could blur all the boundaries between basic and clinical science. Similar to the complex thought required to comprehend a galaxy in a new universe, his mind could grasp the worlds of medical and basic science and see possibilities that no one else saw.

With his immediate goal to save the burned pilot, his first thought was to use tissue culture to expand the available skin. He was pursuing the idea of making what he thought of as a skin soup. He collected spare bits of leftover skin from a plastic surgeon's operations and tried to grow them in tissue culture. Naively, he thought they could be used to seed the raw areas of the burned pilot's skin to generate small islands of tissue to spring up.

Applying the watery creation was frustrating. But he and his plastic-surgeon colleagues applied the "soup" as best they could. They watched and waited and then disappointingly found that none of the epidermal seeds grew.

He went back to the drawing board. His next idea was to *expand* available skin. He froze skin samples and, with a special instrument, cut the tissue into slices a tenth of a millimeter thick. These could then be spread evenly with a fine paintbrush on the wounds.

But again, the seeds did not take.

About this time Peter realized he wasn't doing that poor airman any good at all. Indeed, the burned pilot died of infection. Painfully, Peter realized he had to absorb his failures as lessons from which he could learn.

He moved on to explore the most basic and far-reaching question: how to exchange skin between those who are not closely related without the foreign tissue being rejected. In that answer lay a whole new universe of life-saving possibilities. Despite the allure of pursuing the secrets of the body's exquisite powers of discrimination, he knew the studies would take many years, for he would be unveiling the ultimate understanding of the body's immune system.

Later, he would write: "A scientist who wants to do something original and important must experience, as I did, some kind of shock that forces upon his intention the kind of problem that should be his duty and will become his pleasure to investigate."

Peter's investigative pleasure had taken flight. For the next fourteen years he worked each day and half the night to unlock the biological secrets of how the body recognizes tissue that is borrowed, foreign to itself—all with the end goal of saving lives.

But in that year of 1939, his research would bring no help to the crashed Spitfire pilots; nor would it help Charles, when he lay near death more than five years later. Yet Peter Brian Medawar was onto something.

No one ever doubted that Peter was extraordinary. His biggest surprise, which he himself discovered, was the depth to which he could love.

Six-foot-five and eye-catchingly handsome, he was often the subject of his colleagues' curiosity and veiled envy. As a colleague said, "One could feel that too much was given to one man—handsome, brilliant, charming, a beautiful wife, wonderful children." All agreed he was staggeringly intelligent and "if you played a game of bridge with Medawar's mother, it would become painfully clear where Peter got his IQ."

He met Jean on his twentieth birthday, February 28, 1935. They were both sitting in the same zoology lecture hall at Oxford University. The Oxford system of education, the most extravagant education in the world, assigned a tutor to each student in a one-on-one private system of instruction that starts as soon as a tutor summons his student for an interview. It is then that a subject is chosen for the student to study for a passing grade, equal to a bachelor's degree. When Peter had tried for a scholarship to Oxford University from his public school, he had failed and entered at the age of seventeen for the "Michaelmas" (autumn) term of 1932.

Soon, it became apparent Peter couldn't narrow down a field of interest to study. So, he simply named natural sciences as a catch-all concentration. Drawn to what he considered "the grandeur of the concepts that informed evolution, heredity, epigenesis [the theory that individuals develop from instructions written in the unstructured egg rather than enlarging from a preformed entity], comparative anatomy, anthropology, demography and ecology," his mind was too far-reaching to be corralled into the study of one subject. To simplify his interests for the sake of requirements, he finally said he would "read" zoology.

"Jean Taylor Shinglewood," he later said, "was the most beautiful woman student in Oxford. I fell in love with her, of course, but I did not meet her much socially because I was not a very well-off student and we tended to move in different circles."

That day of his birthday in 1935, when they were both sitting on hardwood benches in the zoology lecture hall, Jean saw that Peter wore a cheap chain-store jacket and a shirt of bright blue knit, obviously chosen because it needed no ironing. "His hair was black and curly and there was a lot of it. When he was thinking he twiddled the front part absentmindedly, making twists which he forgot about. They made him look mildly diabolical."

During the lecture, most students took notes. Peter wrote only a word or two on a piece of paper, then at the end of class, crumpled it up and threw it away. When someone asked him why, he answered, "Because it's all in the textbooks."

It was Jean who made the first move.

As she headed toward him, ready to ask a made-up question as an excuse to speak to him, a classmate caught her and whispered, "I suppose you've heard he's not English. He's got Arab blood, you know."

Missing her timing, she later approached him in the library. She went to where he was sitting and asked in a whisper that he explain the meaning of the word *heuristic* in a book on philosophy she was reading. After he told her, she went back to her place, then realized she had not remembered a bit of what he had told her. Willing to risk looking like a fool, she went back and admitted that she hadn't remembered what he'd told her. Patiently, he whispered again that *heuristic* came from the Greek *eureka*, meaning "I have found it," which also turned out to be their own heuristic moment. From then on, they were rarely separated.

He sported gentlemanly manners, a crisp British accent, a dry, wicked sense of humor, and soon he and Jean were sharing an outlook that Peter called "the human comedy," or "the human predicament." He considered the British class system ridiculous and said that there was only one race of people, the human race. As he watched some interchange between people, or the development of some situation, he'd cut an eye at Jean and utter "RTL"—shorthand for "rich tapestry of life."

When she began spending time with him in his apartment, she saw he had one pan, a gas ring to cook on, and only cheap pats of ground beef. His landlady suspected he smoked opium because his cigarettes smelled odd. Certainly, he looked avant-garde enough to fuel such gossip. About this time, Jean began wondering if she were entering a relationship like the one described in George Eliot's *Middlemarch* between the characters Dorothea Brooke and the dazzling intellectual Mr. Casaubon, with his sterile, prune-dried intellect that would never produce. No doubt Jean was pondering the likely fate of many wives of that period: that she would disappear into her husband's life, known only by his career and accomplishments. Or lack of them. Well, if so, she was willing to take her chances. "I only knew that [Peter] was an uncut diamond, packed with light and fire . . . and I wanted to be with him permanently. Later on, it became obvious and everyone saw it." Indeed, he once admitted that if he had not found Jean, to understand and love him, he would have had a nervous breakdown, unable to commit his energies to science.

He didn't propose. They just knew they never wanted to be separated.

6

Curiosity Awakened

ON THE AFTERNOON that the medical team treating Charles decided to find a skin donor for him as a stopgap measure to save his life, they learned that a young man who worked on one of the wards had died suddenly that morning. His parents lived only twenty miles away. Quickly, one of the team doctors drove there to talk to them, who—when they understood the gravity of Charles's teetering condition and the hope that their son's body might offer—signed the papers to allow the surgical team to use his skin.

Right away, Charles was rushed to the operating room. The allografts harvested from the cadaver were placed on the worst of his burns. One team of surgeons worked on his face, while Joe and another surgeon used tweezers to position little squares of new skin on Charles's hands. To Joe, it felt as if he were planting seeds, preparing the soil to accept and grow the precious pieces of skin.

He also realized that the deformities of Charles's face and hands were worse than any he had ever seen. If the skin grafts worked to save his life, the surgical team would have to spend many months, and even years, giving him a new face and usable hands. But, of course, all that depended on whether the allografts could keep him alive long enough for scar to form. And scarring had its own complications: restricting movement and creating hideous deformities.

Wait and see was their only plan.

Each day Joe studied Charles's wounds and the health of the borrowed skin. He dreaded the day he would see the borrowed skin turn gray and shrink with the first signs of rejection. But on day fourteen, the cadaver skin was still alive. Even beyond day fourteen, the cadaver skin was still spreading. The borrowed skin even held its healthy color.

The allografts taken from the dead boy were lasting longer than any research predicted. *Why?* Why was Charles's body not rejecting the allografts in the usual time? Fascinated, Joe and the treatment team watched as the cadaver skin grafts lasted nearly a month.

This was a scientific phenomenon. A phenomenon that seemed truly miraculous.

Giving rein to his curiosity, Joe's mind spun with questions, possibilities, and theories. And curiosity had always driven his intellect. As a boy in Milford, Massachusetts, he would come upon ants making trails on the paths he walked in the woods. He had always wondered: was the same ant the leader every time? Of course, there was no way to discover *that* answer, but in his adulthood, whenever he saw an ant, he would laugh while remembering his boyhood inquisitiveness. And now, despite the many years that had passed, his curiosity was still the same: once awakened, it refused to be ignored.

The case of Charles's skin grafts was taking root in his memory, returning over and over with a relentless demand for answers. One thing was clear: Charles's body had somehow tricked his immune system. Joe made a list of possibilities: could there be a closer kinship between the tissues of certain unrelated individuals than science could yet identify? Was Charles's body simply too weak to attack the foreign grafts? Even more compelling: if successful skin grafts between identical twins were possible, then why not organs as well?

While there was no scientific explanation for Charles's seemingly miraculous survival, there was, however, an answer to unlock beneath the unexpected survival of the borrowed skin from a boy who had died.

JOE KNEW THE MEDICAL LITERATURE: transplanting tissues between individuals would never be possible. *The Biological Basis of Individuality* by Dr. Leo Loeb discussed the impossibility at length, and some considered his book dogma. As early as the eighteenth century, experimental transplants in humans and animals had been tried, but always the results failed from the biological force that formed a barrier when the body perceived the transplanted tissue to be foreign. The give-and-take of organs was science fiction. Serious consideration of transplanting organs was even labeled crazy.

And there was plenty of evidence to support that view. One need only look at the fantasy figures in art to see how, over the centuries, the human mind played with the idea of transplanting features from one to another. In mythology, the chimera is a female with a lion's head, a goat's body, and a dragon's tail. The Minotaur has a human body and the head of a bull. The Sphinx, a woman's head and a lion's body. Even a mermaid is a grafting of a woman's body and a fish's tail.

For a while, bizarre attempts to borrow the sexual prowess of animals or of other humans became a fad. In Chicago in 1916, Dr. Frank Lydston, eager to regain youth, transplanted slices of human testicles into the scrotum of patients, including his own! Physicians carried out similar rejuvenation dreams using prisoners, claiming to discover what a Viennese sexologist and hormone researcher called "a charm to wean us from the vulgar habit of growing old."

However, the view that transplantation was a half-baked idea, *and* impossible—along with the fact that most of the medical community embraced that view—did not intimidate Joe. He vowed to plunge into what was deemed unfeasible and explore it for himself. The fact that Charles was alive, and his allografts had lasted nearly a month, proved that what was expected was not always the outcome.

While scrubbing for surgery with other young surgeons, Joe began bringing up the subject of tissue transplantation. The conversations were thrilling and heartening. Furthermore, he had his own personal experience to add to the subject. From what he had witnessed with Charles, the idea of sharing organs between two individuals did not seem so great a leap now.

———————

THAT LEAP WOULD soon land in a different world. War was helping to push medicine into a golden age. Desperate measures gave rise to innovation. And innovation was producing a flood of new treatments that were shared across borders, even between countries at war. One of these would later play a significant role in Joe's quest to borrow organs. And, strangely enough, it began with sausage casing and tomato cans—the humble parts used by a young physician in Nazi-occupied Holland as he began to build the first dialysis machine. The fact that he was doing it under the noses of the Nazis made it that much more exciting. Strangely enough, too, it was inspired by the brutal bombings that destroyed cities, crushing thousands of victims.

During the London attacks, when people were dug out of the rubble, alive, it was found that their kidneys had stopped functioning from shock. However, if they could be kept alive for days or weeks, their kidneys often healed and spontaneously recovered, doing their essential job of cleansing the blood, ridding it of wastes in the form of urine. Blood transfusions had been found to be the prime treatment for shock, and since by then the Red Cross had learned how to store blood close to battle sites, many of the crushed victims survived the temporary renal failure that became known as *crush syndrome.*

A new reverence for the resilience of the pair of glands—fist-sized, riding on either side of the spine, shaped like beans, hence the name "kidney bean"—gave rise to the idea of developing a bridge, an artificial kidney of some kind to tide a crushed victim over to that magic hour when their kidneys healed.

In 1938, Willem Kolff, a young doctor at the University of Groningen, was caring for a young man slowly dying from kidney failure. Feeling helpless to relieve his patient's agony, he was further distressed by the boy's mother when he told her that her son would die. She was dressed in Sunday black, with a white lace cap, and in her grief she was inconsolable. Frustrated and distraught, Kolff was suddenly struck with an idea. If he could only dialyze the boy's blood, remove twenty grams of urea and other toxic products, he might relieve his patient's nausea and other symptoms. Saving the boy's life might even be possible.

Right away, Kolff went to a professor of biochemistry, who showed him the wonders of cellophane tubing made from sausage casing. Intrigued, Kolff worked on constructing his idea under the Nazis, who were too ignorant to understand what he was doing. He fiddled with the sausage casing, winding it around tomato cans, then passed the boy's blood across it with salt water on the other side. The idea was that the sausage membrane would cleanse the blood when small molecules passed through. Despite his long hours of working, the boy died. Even though Kolff was unable to save his patient's life, he knew he had an idea worth pursuing.

Failure followed failure. When so many of his other patients died, his professor told him to stop. Kolff didn't stop. He worked on the project whenever his professor was away. His method was labor intensive. After filling the tubing with urea-poisoned blood, he rocked it on a board in a saline bath. After a half hour of dialysis, all the urea had passed out of the blood. In time, he perfected his method when two developments made it successful: heparin, the chemical substance that prevents blood from clotting, and the manufacture of long cellophane tubing to replace the humble sausage casing.

He next built several apparatuses, paying for all the parts himself. None was made well enough to use clinically. Then fate intervened. Kolff's Jewish professor of medicine committed suicide and was replaced by a Dutch Nazi as head of the department. Kolff began making plans to leave. The final push came on May 10, 1940, when he and his wife were on the top floor of the hospital and saw a huge mushroom cloud from bombs dropped by the German Luftwaffe on Rotterdam. They fled to Kampen, a small city in the north. There, he engaged a local company, following his design, to produce a machine that became the first artificial kidney.

Of the fifteen patients he treated in 1943, only one survived, but he had a method to at least relieve suffering. He also wondered if he were not in an occupied country but in the United States would he be more successful.

Undaunted, he built more dialysis machines.

In 1944, he published his findings in a Scandinavian journal, but during the war, Scandinavian literature was not read in America. It would be only after the war that American physicians would learn of what Kolff described in Dutch as an "artificial kidney." In 1945, he saved his first patient and sent what few dialysis machines he had to hospitals in other war-torn countries. His last disappeared behind the Iron Curtain in Poland.

In 1945, Joe was unaware of Kolff's artificial kidney. But his ideas, prompted by Charles's long-lasting borrowed skin, were intersecting with Kolff's innovations. Borrowing a kidney might be another way to extend a patient's life. Even more far-reaching, transplanting organs might lead to a future shift in the treatment of disease.

In only two years, Kolff's and Joe's ideas would come together in Boston at the perfect time with the perfect team of Franny and Peter. First, though, the war would have to end.

PART II

7

"Just Gimme a Coupla Aspirin. I Already Got a Purple Heart"

WITH HIS EYES BANDAGED, Charles relied on hearing voices to know what was happening around him. He marveled that, at times, people talked over him as if he did not exist.

"My God," he heard a nurse say, "I bet he doesn't weigh eighty pounds. He's nothing but bones."

Knowing that by now Miriam had been told of the crash, he listened for footsteps that might be hers. Privately, he was chewing on a worry that he could not mention to anyone. Cycling in his mind, fading in and out with his pain medications, was the scene from a movie he recalled in which a man lives hidden away in Paris wearing a mask because his face is so hideous. After he falls in love with the heroine of the story, he takes off his mask and the girl screams in terror.

When Miriam saw him, would she scream in terror?

And then, "Charles?" The voice was familiar. "Charles?"

On the brink of consciousness, he wanted to identify the voice as hers and said aloud, "Miriam? Is that you?"

He heard only the sound of running feet.

"She'll be right back," a nurse said.

Faint with the shock of seeing him, she had indeed run out of the room. But then, composed, she came back in. Touching his leg, with her voice steady now, she said, "Hello, Charles. It's good to see you."

"I'll be all right now, Miriam. Now that you're here."

She stayed all afternoon. She sat beside him, leaning in, telling him that she had been given rooms nearby. "And they're going to let me stay. I have Freddie with me. We're going to stay in rooms set aside just for us. I can be here every day."

Freddie, now ten months old, was being looked after by one of the other families of patients who were staying in the rooms that Miriam spoke of. What Charles did not know was that those rooms had been set aside for the families of patients expected to die. All around him other injured soldiers were also stoically fighting off death with a studied nonchalance, a favorite expression being, "Just gimme a coupla aspirin. I already got a Purple Heart."

Daily, Charles's dressings were changed and his body chemicals monitored. More cadaver allografts were placed over his burns. But until his life was clearly out of danger, Joe and the other team of surgeons could not consider building him a new face, as well as a pair of hands. First they needed to make him a pair of eyelids. Since his eyes were at risk of infection, and, therefore, blindness, nurses covered them with dressings and antibiotic ointments twenty-four hours a day.

As he lay there, unable to see, but feeling that he was moving past the point of dying, he thought he might begin imagining his future. Moments of his childhood came awake in his memory, in particular one day in spring.

He was five, walking barefoot in the creek that ran in front of the house where he and his older brother Jack lived with their mother. It was in the small Alabama town where he'd been born, and the house, with its gray-weathered wood—a shack, really—

rested on stilts. He could recall the sloshing of the creek between his toes, and the feel of the mud and the way he crawled with Jack under the house to play, building dirt roads and sliding on their bellies like movie cowboys sneaking up on robbers. It was as if he could again smell and feel the dirt, and he remembered vividly hearing a Model T drive up and stop. From under the house, he and Jack watched the legs of a man jump the creek and walk toward the house's rickety steps. They heard him knock at the door. Their mother answered and then the sound of her voice was followed by a haunting silence. The man came down the steps and leaned down to look at them. Their eyes met. He was holding a cardboard box. He coaxed them out. "How old are you, son?" he asked. Charles held up five fingers. Jack said, "Six." "I'm taking you to a nice place to live," he said. "You'll like it there. There are lots of boys your ages there." He led them to the car. Jack cried. Charles looked at his older brother, stunned; Jack never cried. The man ushered them into the backseat of the Model T and drove them to an orphanage with the cardboard box of clothes on the seat beside them. From that day, the family Charles had known was lost to him.

Now Miriam was coming every day, spending hours with him. As he became stronger and the threat of his death receded, she took an apartment in town for herself and Freddie. Each day she came, she told him about the exploits of their toddler. This was the family he had started as his own. Before he had left for the war, he and Miriam had dreamed of having many children. Would she, still? A dread tormented his thoughts. Would Miriam still want the life they had once envisioned?

Other unknowns were eating at him. What would he do with the rest of his life? Would he be able to provide for the large family they had dreamed of? Would he fall into depression and despair, and give up? Would the trauma of the crash become emotionally crippling?

Another more dangerous unknown—private, not to be spoken of—threatened: would Miriam still want him? Would the love knot they had constructed in their youth be enough to make it through *this*?

———

CHARLES'S AMERICA WAS CHANGING. War production was pumping $300 million a day into the economy, making the joblessness of the Great Depression recede like a bad memory. The war that involved 100 million people from more than thirty countries was making America a world power.

The American GI—the initials standing for "General Issue"—was now recognized everywhere as a conquering hero. Yet, the wet-behind-the-ears adolescent who left home frequently came back with dull eyes and the stuff-of-war traumatic despair. The irony was that while the GI became a comic book or TV character portrayed as slightly befuddled and food for laughs, he was actually battle-hardened and haunted. In combat, GIs didn't shave or get their hair cut—not because they wanted to look cool—but because they lacked razors, shaving cream, mirrors, and hot water.

GI suffering was also felt at home: many on the home front sacrificed and suffered the loss of sons, brothers, husbands, and fathers. But the signs that war was good for the American economy were obvious. The famous journalist Edward R. Murrow warned: "We are the only nation in this war which has raised its standard of living since the war began—if hardships do things to the mind, so do comforts."

That January of 1945, when Joe first met Charles, Franklin D. Roosevelt had just been inaugurated for his fourth term. Until 1937, a US president was always inaugurated on March 4, a tradition that FDR was the first to break. And for his fourth term, feeling the effects of post-poliovirus and heart failure, the president stood at the South Portico of the White House to deliver a simple five-minute speech, all the length of time he could stand. Fearing muscle loss in his thumbs, he secretly practiced writing his name to be able to pen his signature in public. Despite his haunting fears that the poliovirus that had struck him twenty-four years before was returning to claim the rest of him, he had been successful in assuring the American people he was fit to bring the war to a close.

And he was determined not just to end the war but to prevent all others. His dream to establish an organization, among what he called global neighbors, to hash out their differences was becoming a reality. The United Nation's first meeting was set for that next April. First, though, he needed to end the war, and to do so by preventing his greatest nightmare, which his joint chiefs had predicted. They warned that invading Japan would extend the war into 1946 and cost the lives of up to a million Americans.

To avoid that nightmare, he beguiled and humored the brutal Russian dictator, Joseph Stalin, by calling him "Uncle Joe," getting him to promise to join the Allies to fight Japan within two months of the surrender of Germany. He also got Stalin to agree that Russia would become part of the United Nations, the organization he passionately engineered while president as an instrument for keeping peace. And he was excited to attend its first meeting as its first American delegate that late April in San Francisco.

It would be a meeting he would not live to see.

Nor would he witness the cosmic force unleashed on Japan at the end of that summer.

Since October 1939, Roosevelt had known of the possibility of a bomb so powerful it could end the war. But atomic scientists were a breed of their own; few understood what they studied or even how to pronounce *nuclear physicist*.

It was a German-Jewish female scientist, Lise Meitner, who, in March 1938, was bombarding uranium with neutrons in a laboratory in Berlin, when she found astonishing results that led to understanding what unleashing the universe's power could mean in making a bomb. With such a weapon, Hitler could rule the world or destroy it. As Hitler's men came after Lise, she fled to Sweden, settling near the esteemed physicist Niels Bohr.

Soon German physicists began migrating to America. And, in a comic twist, just before Bohr escaped to America, he poured some of his heavy water—necessary for slowing down neutrons to release nuclear power—into a large beer bottle and put it in his refrigerator. There it would sit through five years of Nazi rule.

On January 16, 1939, Bohr received a telegram from Lise describing how she and an assistant had split an atom, freeing 200 million volts of electricity. It was then that Bohr and other physicists predicted that if uranium could be harnessed, it could be twenty million times as powerful as TNT. That was when two physicists decided to warn the president.

Since they didn't have access to FDR, they went to see Einstein, who, shuffling in slippers, answered the door. When he heard why they had come, he said that the possibility of a chain reaction in uranium had not occurred to him, but, realizing the danger of Hitler having physicists capable of producing an atomic bomb, he wrote a letter to Roosevelt.

When the letter arrived, the president, eating breakfast, asked an aide to read it to him. Understanding the threat posed by such a massive bomb being built in Germany, Roosevelt said, "What you are after is to see that the Nazis don't blow us up." And so the war took on another dimension.

The public knew nothing of the prospect of an atomic bomb. Few *did* know. But for those who did, it became imperative that America get the bomb before Hitler. While it was easy to understand what harnessing the power of the universe as a weapon of war could mean, there were others eager to understand the new science that had been unveiled for purposes of good.

Among those would be Joe Murray and Franny Moore, who, ten years later, would begin exploring the use of nuclear radiation to break the age-old barrier of rejection in a desperate patient brave enough to borrow an organ. But until then, the step-by-step development of the bomb would shift into a world trying to understand what science had unveiled.

———

SOON AFTER PETER and Jean met and were still getting to know each other, Jean, though completely attracted to him and totally in love with him, could not help wondering about his character. Was he solid? Could he be counted on?

A major test came one night in his apartment when she became sick. Trying to cover up her nausea, she failed to overcome it and, much to her horror, threw up in his one and only skillet. Peter gently hustled her into a taxi back to her college dorm. Furthermore, he never mentioned her embarrassing moment, which she knew had come from drinking too much wine. The next morning, she knew that *yes*, he was brilliant, but he was also sound: he could be relied upon in a crisis. She also knew she had found her life's calling: to take care of him and to help him succeed as the brilliant scientist he seemed destined to be.

But there were problems with her family accepting him. His dark complexion and thick curly hair often led to suspicions that he was not English and therefore unsuitable for Jean. When Peter explained that his mother was Edith Muriel Dowling, a quite wonderful English woman, and his father was Nicholas Medawar, a Lebanese businessman, the facts made little difference.

Of course, Jean married Peter anyway. When her source of income from her family was cut off, she didn't care. From almost the moment she met Peter, she dedicated her life to him, gladly and completely.

Born a twin, Jean was the one to survive, becoming the oldest of three daughters of an American mother and an English father, a physician who, by the time Jean met Peter, was very frail. Perhaps being the sole survivor of twins, she was raised with a sense of destiny and the confidence to go with it. Soon after she met Peter, she convinced him to take an examination "for honors" at the end of his studies. Not only did she know he was brilliant enough to catch up, but the accomplishment would come with a graduate student stipend that would help them to marry.

What taught her even more about Peter was a crisis that came near the end of the two years they had known each other. She was supposed to produce some kind of respectable research to be awarded a BS degree. Panicked, because she had set up a hypothesis to discover the function of lymphocytes, generally known as white blood cells, she despaired that the work was not coming together. Already, it was known that white blood cells poured into the blood every day, but their numbers in the circulation did not increase. Why? She was trying to find out if primitive white blood cells developed from other white blood cells, or had a special function of their own. The new and complicated universe of the immune system was being studied from many angles, and Jean, although daunted by the complexities, was adding her part—even if slight.

Of course, it didn't hurt that she was being driven by fear that she would not graduate without a written thesis, so she worked relentlessly and with constant panic. Her lab was next to Peter's in the pathology building. And he, sensing her distress, came forward. Not only did he guide her as she wrote her thesis, but he also typed the whole shebang at blistering speed—with two fingers. He saved her. And furthermore, he never teased her about her panic or the fact that she squeaked past the requirements of a degree.

In the following months, as their relationship deepened, tiffs started. In what Peter called interruptions to their "being the greatest of friends," he had to sort out their feelings, which he did rather bluntly. He realized that when Jean was badgering him to pay attention to something she wanted to show him and he didn't look up or listen, she became upset. He realized his obsessiveness and apologized, telling her, "You have first claim on my love, but not on my time." This later led to Jean's tactic of asking, "Peter, are you thinking?" If he said *yes*, she did not talk. Other times, she would pull his arm and say, "Look, Peter, *do* look," and he would glance at whatever it was rather than look, smile at her, and say, "Yesss—lovely." Then he would go back to thinking.

In time, when Jean fully understood the value of the work he was doing, she could then laugh at his obsessive ways. Always, their strongest bond was a "hopeful attitude in life, faith in what science might achieve, and a deep commitment to each other." Embracing the French poet Saint-Exupéry's view that "Love does not consist of gazing at each other, but in looking outward together in the same direction," they set the date for their wedding.

Two days before Peter's twenty-second birthday, they married in the Oxford Registry Office, then followed it up with a sherry party in their Banbury Road flat. Soon, Jean began to savor a joke on him as they set up housekeeping. If a spider got into the house from the garden and sat looking down at them from the ceiling, she would ask him what kind it was and then tease him that she was living with a zoology genius who couldn't identify anything. It was she who had to catch the specimen and return it to the garden.

In those early months of their marriage, when she had sudden pangs of worrying about how deep his regard for her went—brought on mostly by seeing his many women friends, all of whom clearly adored him—she soon realized she was being foolish. *She* was his passion. His work was his life. There was no time, or desire, for anything else.

He had found his calling, and nothing could prevent him from answering the needs of his work, not even Jean. Indeed, in their long-married life of fifty years, there would be many more crises for him than for her. But from the very earliest moments, their bond was strong and deep, never to be broken.

With the war as the canvas for their early married life, Peter's research was urgent. Dedicated to finding a way to treat Spitfire pilots who bailed out of their burning planes, he knew first he had to find out what went on inside grafts of donated skin before he could come up with a treatment. He kept asking: if blood can be transfused, why can't skin be exchanged? The War Wounds Committee gave him a grant, and he left home for two months to work in the burns unit of Glasgow Royal Infirmary. Jean and their young daughter stayed in Oxford, while he moved into a low-rate hotel on the streetcar line to the infirmary. There, he teamed up with a Scottish plastic surgeon, Tom Gibson.

A badly burned older woman came into the infirmary. She had fallen onto her gas fire with injuries so severe, her life was hanging by a thread. Since her brother was willing to supply enough skin for grafting, Peter knew he would now be able to study foreign grafts from a close relative as they were rejected.

Surgeon Tom Gibson covered her wounds with tiny patches of her brother's skin, as well as skin from the woman herself. At regular intervals, he removed one graft from each site to examine under a microscope. Peter set up a workbench in the pathology department to prepare the graft samples himself—an arrangement that suited his restless quest for answers.

After only a few days, he saw that both grafts, the one from the patient and those from her brother, looked very much the same. Yet, after a few more days, the grafts began to look different. Those from her brother were invaded by the white blood-borne cells known to attack an intruder into the body. It was then natural for Peter to test the fate of a second set of donor grafts after the first had been rejected.

Both he and Gibson theorized that the second set from her brother would not survive as long as the first set. And they were right. Immediately, the second set of donor grafts were set upon and destroyed. Furthermore, Peter and the surgeon saw blood vessels invading the graft, a sign of inflammation that impaired the healing process. Ordinarily, inflammation is a useful immune system reaction to help fight infections as small blood vessels dilate to increase blood flow to a site. However, when the body becomes somehow confused and attacks itself with chronic inflammation, serious conditions develop, such as in autoimmune diseases. For the first time, Peter had unveiled a biological force signaling the body to attack a tissue perceived to be foreign. It was the same specific adaptive response as the one that leads to the elimination of bacteria or viruses, organisms foreign to the body.

Most importantly, Peter had illuminated the body's powers of defense. This was significant science that would be known as the "second set" phenomenon. A decade later, this finding would be monumental to Joe and Franny in their attempts to transplant an organ and bypass rejection, for it suggested that the rejection process acted very similarly to an allergic response. And, indeed, if rejection was an immunological process similar to the body recognizing an allergy, then couldn't it be potentially manipulated?

As far back as Louis Pasteur's work in the late 1870s, it was known that something foreign could invade cells. But when Pasteur discovered general bacteria—to be called "germs," from the Latin *germen* meaning *offshoot*—medical practice began to embrace protecting the human body against germs, which was enough of a world-shaking discovery for Pasteur to become known as the "Father of Modern Medicine." From that moment, the practice of medicine changed. Instruments were sterilized in boiling water, and general hygiene was valued and adopted.

Ten years later, Russian zoologist Élie Metchnikoff looked into a microscope at a water flea and saw amoeba-like cells eating vegetable matter, which reminded him of pus, a discovery that pushed the knowledge of disease even further. He designed other studies to show white blood cells assaulting and digesting disease germs. Metchnikoff turned his observations into a cellular view of resistance, likening it to the body's ability to form an army to "fight infection." And the idea of white blood cells took off.

Now Peter's study of the burned woman's borrowed skin grafts proved that the immune system had something akin to a memory. The system could recall a previous invader. It was a simple yet mysterious reaction, and Peter had illuminated the science that had mystified observers for hundreds of years when some fell sick in epidemics while others didn't. Somehow the body remembered the first attack, built weapons against the intruder, and recognized and repelled it swiftly when it tried to invade a second time.

In a sense, Peter had discovered that the human body has not just one brain, but two, the second being the immune system acting in concert to protect well-being, all in the name of survival. He had put the principles of the body's defense on display, and, right away, he and his surgeon coauthor Tom Gibson published their results in 1943 in the *Journal of Anatomy* in an article titled "The Fate of Skin Homografts in Man."

Only one year later, on that fateful day in December 1944, Charles would be so horribly burned that Joe, as a young surgeon with a leaning toward basic science, would naturally be keeping up with current literature. And Peter's findings would inspire his own ideas as he contemplated the idea of borrowing organs, especially skin. Innovative treatments to save the lives of burned pilots arriving daily at Valley Forge were constantly of interest. And Peter's publication was earth-shaking. Joe noted that until then, Dr. James Barrett Brown's observation in St. Louis in 1937 that skin between identical twins could be shared without rejection was the only ray of light in the problem of tissue and organ replacement. But now "with Gibson and Medawar's clear description of the second set phenomenon, the rejection process was seen to be not immutable; instead it implied an allergic or immunological process which potentially might be manipulated."

In other words, tricking the body to accept a foreign tissue now seemed possible.

Soon, Peter and Tom Gibson's work of the second set phenomenon would also be known as *acquired immunity*. This groundbreaking view made it clear that skin tissue from an unrelated donor, even from one closely related, was rejected because the body perceived it *not* of itself, but as that of a foreign invader. Furthermore, the body would even remember it if it were grafted another time. This ability was indeed what Peter liked to refer to as the body's exquisite power of memory.

And it was revolutionizing science. For hundreds of years the problem of rejection was believed to be insoluble. Breaking the rejection barrier was viewed as being no more possible than changing one's blood group. Peter had revised that belief. He had now taken his first step in establishing a new field of science: immunogenetics.

To Joe and Franny, who wanted to explore transplanting organs, Peter's findings were especially encouraging. His large mind was stretching the minds of others, throwing open doorways into the possible.

Yet Peter's most difficult work was ahead. He now had to duplicate and expand his findings as well as explore the possibility of manipulating the body's power of rejection. The next years would be the most intense studies he had ever undertaken, especially since there were no trained technicians to call upon.

In time, the answers would all be with rabbits, mice, cows, and Czechoslovakian chickens.

8

"The Rest Is All Decorations"

LATE IN THE WINTER OF 1945, Joe began constructing Charles a pair of eyelids. With the team of other surgeons, he slit the scar contractures that had formed above Charles's eyes, releasing the scarred skin to fall over his eyeball itself. Then, a new technique to treat similar war wounds had become the treatment of choice for all burned soldiers—to take skin from around the collarbone to create new eyelids. The skin there was a good color match and was also pliable, making it a suitable substitute to protect the eyes.

One day, when Miriam arrived just as the reconstructive surgery was about to start, and his eyes were still bandaged, Charles was startled. "Hey. I didn't hear you come in."

"I know," she said. "I heard the doctor say they're ready to start working on your face. That's a good sign. In a little while you'll be good as new."

"Maybe. But I don't think I'll look like much, Miriam. For one thing, I don't think I'll have any ears. Somewhere, probably in Calcutta, I heard somebody say they had been burned off."

"Oh heck, honey," said Miriam. "You can hear, can't you? That's what ears are for anyway. The rest is all decorations."

In these early surgeries, Joe and the team used general anesthesia. But in the midst of one operation, Charles's heart stopped, and restarting it was so difficult that the team worried about using general anesthesia in the future. For other surgeries, they used only local anesthesia to reduce risk, and the suffering that Charles underwent was unimaginable. Even though the surgeries were mercifully short, Charles moaned for hours afterward. Refusing to ask for more pain medication for fear of becoming addicted, he prided himself on asking for only four shots of morphine a day, when six had been prescribed. His willpower became legend.

A month after Charles's eyes had been repaired, Joe and the team focused on scars around his mouth. After each of the operations, Charles knew he could not eat for a week and gritted his teeth through the pain and vowed he would never risk becoming addicted to painkillers.

Resorting to an ancient technique to treat soldiers with facial war wounds, the Valley Forge team used the same plan to make Charles a nose. It was a technique used in the 1500s in Italy when a common punishment for crimes was to slice off the offender's nose. Ancient surgeons with compassion for those who suffered this harsh act learned to reconstruct noses by borrowing skin from the upper arms. By attaching skin from an arm to the center of a face to keep the blood flow nourishing the tissue, stalks called *pedicles* grew from an arm onto the face. When the pedicle established its own blood supply, it was cut away, leaving a mass of skin from which a nose could be constructed.

There Charles was: his arm connected to his face and unable to move it away for twenty-two days.

———

IN APRIL 1945, President Roosevelt began whispering to his closest confidants that the war would be over by the end of May. The status of the atomic bomb was still uncertain and did not weigh in his calculations. He knew troop strengths, where each army was, and that Allied forces were moving on Berlin. On the afternoon of April 12, while he was at his "Little White House" in Warm Springs, Georgia, for the Easter holiday, he was struck with a cerebral hemorrhage. By 3:35 he was dead.

Two weeks later, Hitler committed suicide. Two weeks after that, Germany surrendered.

VE Day celebrations took place across the world. But injured soldiers still kept coming to Valley Forge. Joe knew he would not be discharged any time soon; indeed, wounded men would trickle in for years.

The focus now was war in the Pacific. But with the end of the war seeming certain, Joe took a few days off in June to travel to Hinmans Corners, New York, where he would marry Bobby Link in St. Christopher's Catholic Church.

As a young girl, Virginia Link walked around the house singing—her operatic voice full and melodic even as a child—so her family called her "Bobolink" after the songbird, a nickname that cleverly included her family's name. Her uncle was the inventor of the flight simulator known as the Link Trainer, and her father, George, ran the Link Aviation Company. Bobby had grown up around creative, driven, and gifted people, which would stand her in good stead when Joe began spending long hours in the operating room and in his lab as he pursued the goal of borrowing organs. Eventually "Bobolink" was simply shortened to "Bobby."

She was an only child, and rather than go to college, she aimed for a music career. Moving to a boarding house in Cambridge, Massachusetts, she studied with master vocalists who would refine her soprano voice. She also studied with pianists to expand her keyboard skills.

She was five years younger than Joe, charming, with striking green eyes, brown hair, and an athletic figure that she put to impressive use on a tennis court (her game was described as "fierce"). Joe's winning her had not been easy. He'd had to draw on his deep well of sweet stubbornness to outlast the competition.

An unwritten rule among his Harvard Medical School friends said that they did not move in on each other's dates. So for a long while Joe had to admire Bobby from a distance. He met her the night when he and several classmates took up an entire row at a Boston Symphony Orchestra concert.

Since they had all been drafted right after Pearl Harbor, they were dressed in their military uniforms. Some had dates, and Joe ended up sitting next to Bobby. That night she was with Joe's classmate, Al Meyer, dressed in his gold-braided naval ensign uniform that made Joe's army khaki's look like a dull sparrow. Again, Joe regretted that the navy had turned him down because of his weak eyesight, giving him now another handicap of having to wear army brown while Al Meyer sat next to Bobby in dazzling navy white.

Taken with Bobby's vivaciousness, Joe stole glimpses of her. He memorized her attractive face. He adored the playful glint in her eyes. During intermission, he maneuvered next to her to strike up a conversation. When he learned that she was a serious music student, he said he was, too, and even told her that he'd studied piano. A moment later, he confessed, admitting his lack of talent, and added that his teacher must have needed the money desperately to take him on.

When he went back to his room in the medical school barracks, he told his roommate he had met the girl he would marry. There was one problem, though: Al.

Weeks later at a group picnic, as friends were singing and drinking beer, Joe and Bobby ended up resting against each other's backs. The feeling of that touch opened a door into what might be, for both of them. After medical school graduation, Al left for St. Louis for his internship and Joe stayed in Boston, tackling his internship at the Peter Bent Brigham Hospital. The chance to win Bobby was now open for the taking—*if* he could pull it off.

Living in a tiny room at the top of Peter Bent Brigham called the Crow's Nest, he checked the mail every day for his active duty assignment. Meanwhile he was gaining as many months of surgical training as he would be allowed. For weeks, he picked up a phone in a lab to call Bobby. But when he asked her out, she always said, "I'm sorry, Joe, I'm busy." Overhearing his conversation, the lab staff turned his rejections into a running joke. But Joe's persistence paid off. He kept asking until he and Bobby hit upon a time they were both free.

On that date, and for several afterward, Bobby didn't even know his last name. She kept calling him Joe Murdock.

That spring, just before he was assigned to Valley Forge, he and Bobby walked along the Charles River. As they talked, their conversation changed. To Joe it seemed a mystery how they managed to reveal their inner selves to each other. He kissed her for the first time in the Arnold Arboretum.

She began visiting him at the hospital. Often he was so tired from working around the clock as an intern, he was dull company. But she kept coming, patiently waiting until he had time to spend with her. Once, while she was watching Joe play tennis in the yearly Mass General - Brigham match, the hospital president assumed she was his wife. Embarrassed, Bobby corrected him, but the possibility stayed.

Until Joe was assigned to his army post, he didn't feel free to commit to a longer relationship. However, in that summer of 1944, when Bobby went home to her family's farm in Binghamton, New York, the letters they wrote back and forth revealed a seriousness they were both ready to admit. In one letter, Bobby brought up the subject of their religious differences. Joe was Roman Catholic; Bobby, Episcopalian. Clearly, she was thinking long term, even in the uncertainty of war.

That fall, after receiving his assignment to report to Valley Forge, he was on his way there when he turned the car toward Bobby's parents' farm, ten miles outside of Binghamton. When he drove up, her mother was in the farmhouse kitchen making a chocolate pie.

No one yet knew that Joe, as a kid, would buy a small can of Hershey's syrup for a nickel and drink it straight up. Nor that even now, as a twenty-five-year-old surgeon, he would pour chocolate syrup on a bowl of cereal—preferring it to coffee—as part of his morning ritual.

In Bobby's family's kitchen that day, he commented only on how good Bobby's mother's pie smelled; also on how much he looked forward to eating a piece. Then, while it baked, he invited Bobby to take a walk.

It was a crystal-clear autumn day. Leaves were at the peak of their color, tinting the woods with red and gold. Soon, Joe and Bobby found themselves standing on a hill overlooking the Chenango River. They sat down to watch a train puff up the valley in the distance, and for a few moments, they sat in silence. Calmly and naturally, they looked at each other and knew it was time. They decided to marry. Yes, it was wartime. But at least now Joe had active duty pay. Yes, the future was uncertain. But this felt right.

When they walked back to the house, Bobby served Joe a piece of her mother's chocolate pie. Then another. She even promised to get the recipe.

Later, when Bobby saw Joe eating cereal with chocolate syrup poured over it, she knew the pie had clinched the deal.

A few days before their wedding, set for June 2, 1945, Joe woke early. He bent over the sink in his small Valley Forge cottage, eating his usual breakfast—a piece of burnt toast with the top layer scraped off. Then he drove to Hinmans Corners, the small town near Bobby's family farm. There, in St. Christopher's Catholic Church, dressed in his uniform, he watched Bobby walk toward him in a long satin dress with a veil. Only family and friends were with them, but the cake was big—even though it wasn't chocolate—and the mood was joyous. After a few days in Atlantic City, Joe brought Bobby to his little rented house among the rolling hills of Pennsylvania.

Even with Germany's surrender, there were still many injured coming from Europe, and doctors were also still needed overseas. Occasionally, Bobby accompanied Joe to the hospital to change dressings and visit patients. Together, they focused on enjoying every moment as the prospect of Joe being reassigned hovered over them, coloring every second. Within a day's notice, one of the surgeons or medical officers would disappear, assigned overseas.

Despite that threat, Joe concentrated on adding to his surgical skills. And, slowly, he realized he was changing. A new interest was catching his attention, one he had never really considered. A seed was being planted that only twenty years later would rearrange his surgical life. Partly it would grow from taking care of Charles. Building Charles a face and hands to wear out into the world was one of the most satisfying privileges he had ever been given.

Soon, Joe and Bobby's first child, Ginny, was on her way. Like most young American couples, they hoped to have a big family. So much of a generation was disappearing in the horrors of war.

In one of those mysteries of coincidence, about which the universe refuses to even give hints, Ginny, that first child that Joe and Bobby would have while at Valley Forge, would be asked one day to turn over her room to a hulking scientist named Peter Medawar while he consulted with Joe and Franny in the new universe of transplantation. No doubt later Peter would put that coincidence in his mental file entitled the *Rich Tapestry of Life.*

9

Please Airdrop One First-Rate Artificial Leg

CHARLES'S HANDS PRESENTED a particular challenge. In reconstructing them, Joe learned the difference between fine and gross surgical techniques. Knowing when to use one or the other required judgment. The most experienced surgeon on the team guided him by saying, "Just try to release all of those bones and tendons that are entrapped by scar. Create as much raw surface as you can. Give as much motion as possible."

Since Charles had lost the tips of all his fingers and both thumbs, Joe did his best to create finger-like structures from the bones and muscles on Charles's palms. Then Joe covered the exposed surfaces with skin taken from wherever he could find a viable donor site.

The months of recuperation for Charles were long—well over a year, and there was still more surgery to do.

As Joe worked to reconstruct Charles, he came to realize that Charles was living proof that a will to survive can overcome enormous odds—and proof that there was great value in reconstructing deformities. Aware of his budding interest in plastic surgery, Joe knew he was being drawn to a road less traveled. Plastic surgery was generally looked down upon by other surgeons, who thought it was mostly cosmetic fixes and, therefore, frivolous. First described in 1818 in Germany, the word "plastic" was used with "repair" to detail treatments of the nose when they were often destroyed by the use of mercury, a treatment for syphilis.

But now, more than a century later, plastic surgery had other uses, and, as Joe looked at the devastation of what the fiery crash had done to Charles's face and hands, he knew he was being led to blend intellectual challenge with the desire to connect with a life dealing with the hardest of tests. To walk out into the world causing others to stare in discomfort, if not horror, had to be terrifying.

In the psyche of each human is the fear of monsters, but the fear of *being* the monster may be even worse. During the months upon months of building Charles a new face and set of hands, Joe wondered if *he* were Charles would he have had the will to survive with nearly all of his body burned? While no wound is as socially devastating as a facial wound, no loss of function is as mentally devastating as taking away the use of hands—especially for a pilot.

He considered "reconstructing Charles" far more than a job; it was a privilege. With his rigorous schedule leaving him little time to contemplate his own life, Joe was seeing that molding, transforming, and artfully crafting tissues to save and improve a life would be a valuable future for a surgeon. He wanted to be part of that.

And always beneath the day-to-day work was the recurring refrain of what he had felt in that early moment when he had seen Charles's first borrowed skin grafts lasting longer than predicted. He had witnessed a scientific phenomenon. That moment was planted deep in his awareness. The fantasy-like idea of transplanting organs was not one to be dismissed.

When the chief of plastic surgery at Valley Forge noticed that Joe spent almost all day and night in the wards, he approached their army supervisor and asked that Joe *not* be sent overseas. Keeping Joe there was proving to be very valuable.

———————

AFTER NINE MONTHS of reconstruction, Charles's eyes were healed to where his bandages could be removed. First off, he asked a nurse for a hand mirror. She said she did not have one. Every nurse he then asked said she did not have one either, *sorry*. Though he found their answers hard to believe—and even after he watched them root around in their purses and still say *no*—he didn't push. He figured they were trying to be kind. His private worry of wondering what his face would eventually look like could not be talked about.

Finally, he dragged himself to the bathroom and looked in the mirror there.

What Charles saw was not what Joe saw. Always, Joe had been able to envision what he could do for Charles, the face he would eventually be able to give him. But what Charles saw that day in the bathroom mirror was alarming. In the patches of skin that had been sewn over his burns, somewhat like a country quilt, there was a tiny hole that was his mouth. There was a mound of flesh for a nose that, he thought, resembled a three-year-old's attempt with modeling clay. As he came out of the bathroom, he said nothing. He went to his bed, curled up, and went to sleep.

The next day, he reveled in the magic of sight. Even though his face was still in the middle of construction, at least he could see. From his hospital room window he studied the expansive grounds, green in late summer, the grass leading into a forest. He liked to watch the trees, their response to breezes, their bending to weather. Everything was as if he had never seen it before.

Every morning he studied the triangle of light coming through the window onto the hardwood floor. He put the ball of his bandaged hand on the window, turned, and studied the two straight-backed chairs and a dresser. He picked up the framed picture of Miriam and Freddie and held it between his bandaged hands.

He was becoming someone he never imagined he would be—not only in the way he looked, but in the way he had to think. It was almost time to take his first walk out into the world. He wanted to see his son.

Toward that goal, with Miriam's help, he began leaving his room. The world of Valley Forge, with its patients, doctors, nurses, attendants, visitors, office and work crews, gave him a makeshift substitute for what he would eventually see, and who would see him. He needed to learn how to handle that. He needed to learn how to react without flinching at the looks of awe and pity. On the other hand, he knew that his appearance could also lift the spirits of parents and wives as he passed them in the corridors. Being as courageous in life as in the cockpit of a war plane was now his job.

He'd been immobile for twenty-six months. His legs were unsteady. With his hands still in balls of bandages that looked like boxing gloves, it would be disastrous if he stumbled and fell. He could not risk breaking a bone in his fragile hands. For that reason, he was not allowed to walk alone.

With Miriam's help, he began visiting other patients on the floor, stopping to chat. All liked to recall their escapes from danger: a stalled airplane, a jammed gun, an undetonated grenade. Near misses became funny in retrospect. They even made stories out of the actions that had brought them there, maimed and scarred. They talked of war as if they had been spectators, not participants. They made it all seem as if it had happened long ago and far away.

At the end of the hall was Charles's favorite place, a ward with many pilots—that rare breed of men who are never still for long. They yelled jokes from bed to bed. They wheeled up and down the corridors as if they were ten-year-old boys loose on the streets of a neighborhood, trying to race, yelling dares beyond the hearing of the nurses. With no air conditioning and no such thing as television, discomfort and boredom didn't exist. Card tables were set up in the corners. Poker games went on for hours, with the injured men hiding their winnings from the nurses. Stories flowed, always a bit outrageous, always humorous.

One favorite was of an ace Allied pilot who'd been shot down by the Germans and lost a leg in the crash. When the Germans shot him down again and found that his artificial leg had been damaged in *that* crash, his captors sent word to an Allied Air Force unit to *please airdrop a new prosthesis.*

The hijinks never waned. Injured men yelled jokes between beds; they thought up games and competitions to carry out in wheelchairs or on stretchers.

One day as Charles was on his walk about in the hospital, he saw a group of patients collected around a dignified elderly woman reading her poetry. "Who's that?" Miriam asked the ward attendant standing near the door.

"We're calling her the *poetry lady*. She just came in and said she was from Philadelphia and was going to make the boys happy by reading her poetry to them."

"Is it any good?" Charles asked.

"You see where I am, don't you," said the orderly. "I was sneaking out when you came in."

Soon, men on crutches and others in wheelchairs were scooting out until the poetry lady sat all alone beside a boy trapped in his bed by a leg in traction. As Charles and Miriam walked toward them, the eyes of the young man shot them an SOS.

Walking closely up to the poet, Charles said, "I was thinking that with all the boys in the Naval Hospital in Philly, you could read to the boys there without traveling so far."

How kind he was to think of them, she said.

Over the next weeks, when she kept coming, an injured soldier picked up on Charles's suggestion and wrote to her pretending to be a soldier in another hospital. He said he had heard her poetry was so beautiful and compelling, would she please consider entertaining the men at the other hospital across town?

Cleverly, he arranged to have his letter postmarked from that very town.

The story of the poetry lady became a favorite, not just for its humor but also for the kindness with which the problem had been solved.

Since their ages were much the same, the barrier that might have otherwise existed in the relationship between patient and doctor was relaxed. It was not that the young injured men discarded their high regard for the medical staff taking care of them, it was just that their sense of fun did not get in the way, either. The atmosphere they created at Valley Forge was exceptional and contagious. And Joe recognized that.

The musical *Oklahoma!* had just come out, sweeping the country with its charm. Often, when off duty, a young doctor would start singing, "All the cattle are standing like statues . . ." and others would quickly join in. Joe and Bobby always added their voices. Despite his eagerness to be discharged from the army and back to his surgical training in Boston, Joe savored his moments at Valley Forge. He recognized that a civilian hospital would never be like this. The place was special; the time was unique. The horror of war demanded close bonding, the lessening of boundaries, and an unbridled emphasis on fun.

Even with Germany's surrender, the medical needs in Europe were staggering. Throughout the winter of 1945, casualties continued to trickle in. To care for them, and for the German prisoners of war housed there, the staff had to stay in place. The surgeon general declared those surgeons with extensive plastic surgery experience to be essential. Among these was Joe.

His military status was frozen. Promoted to major, he felt the reward meager, for he was now in a holding pattern. His greatest worry was that in Boston the general surgery residencies would be taken by the time he was discharged. Those positions were competitive. He could miss his chance.

―――――――

WHILE FRANNY WAS stretching his talents into the new universe of twentieth-century medicine, Joe was caught in the aftermath of war. Charles was adjusting to the new life he would lead, and Peter was dug in, spending night and day in his laboratory, pushing, prodding, designing some of the most elegant scientific experiments yet known for biology to give up its secrets.

Peter was indeed a strange sight on the Oxford campus. Often someone would look, and then look again to realize that what they were really seeing was an extraordinarily tall man loping across the campus carrying a rabbit. Peter took care of his research rabbits himself and carried them from the animal house to his laboratory. Italian prisoners of war were assigned to be in charge of the research animals at Oxford, but Peter didn't quite trust them, so he cleaned all the rabbits' cages himself and fed them. With no trained technicians to call on to help him, he also operated on all the animals himself.

To duplicate his findings of the second set phenomenon, he spent months cutting and staining the microscopic sections. He photographed them on the scale necessary to create accurate documentation. The work was grueling. Since it was at the height of the war, Peter felt his work was the least he could do for the war effort. Compared to what men had to put up with in the North African desert and in the battlefields of Europe, his work seemed a picnic. After working long hours, he felt downright guilty if he went home at night without a briefcase full of material to be read before the next morning.

His schedule included serving as a warden on air-raid duty in north Oxford. With him those nights was J. R. R. Tolkien, the eventual author of *The Lord of the Rings*, whom Peter found delightfully learned and charming. They each wore heavy overcoats on cold and rainy nights, and Peter rode a bicycle on duty—one that had such a small mechanism attaching the pedals to the wheels that, as he pedaled, he went hardly anywhere—while Tolkien stood watching, chattering comically, comparing him to an inept messenger.

Peter spent long hours in his lab each day carrying out his research design. He gave twenty-five rabbits a skin graft from one of the others, adding up to a total of six hundred grafts. Then he watched and waited, hoping to unlock a way to give burned soldiers borrowed skin grafts that would not be rejected.

He tended carefully to his laboratory rabbits, keeping detailed records day by day as all the grafts sloughed off, rejected. This elaborate procedure proved clearly that, with rabbits as a research model, an immunity-provoking factor was responsible for rejecting donated skin from an unrelated donor. This discovery was crucial. It was a substantial scientific finding, and he published it right away. Then he quickly went on with other experiments.

By today's standards, his research tools were primitive. He explored various side roads, one of which was investigating the phenomenon of pigment spread. Thinking that spotted black-and-white guinea pigs and Friesian cattle become parti-colored animals by their dark pigmentation "infecting" their counterparts in pale skin, he designed experiments to test his theory.

He hypothesized that the pale skin received a signal to manufacture dark pigmentation. After putting skin grafts of dark skin into a pale area, he waited to see the reaction. Two years later, he finally had to admit that his idea had been mistaken.

Rating his failure as an occupational hazard of the scientific life, he turned to another study and took comfort in knowing that the scientist too scared to speculate boldly can hardly have a creative life at all. He said that such a scientist would end up as "one of those sad, sterile men of letters whose taste is so refined and judgment so nice that they cannot bring themselves to the point of putting pen to paper."

If there was one thing that Peter lacked, it was not creativity, or its handmaiden, boldness. Always keeping up on research in other countries, he kept an eye on other scientists undertaking the question of how individuals might share tissues, which could then be applied to transplanting kidneys in patients dying of renal failure. Crush syndrome from the London bombings was a lingering nightmare, as well as a prod for scientific study. New understandings of the workings of the human body were enthralling. Hope for saving lives was letting in new light for more and more experiments and more and more innovative treatments.

Transplant studies in various countries were especially helpful for those driving hard toward pioneering the first successful transplant. And Peter took all that information and kept it close at hand.

That other war, the one across continents, was pushing another type of scientific exploration—the one to find the most deadly weapon to end the worldwide conflict.

———

HAVING INHERITED THE LIKELIHOOD of losing up to a million American lives invading Japan, and the potential option of ending the war before an invasion, President Truman asked to review his choices. On April 24, the secretary of war walked into the Oval Office to give a complete briefing on the Manhattan Project, which was producing what was called the "gadget."

As the president was listening, he stood up. When the briefing was finished, he abruptly sat down. This was not the choice he was hoping for. Pointing out that the use of atomic energy should not simply be considered in terms of military weapons, his advisors emphasized that understanding how to harness nuclear power meant "a new relationship to the universe." They stressed that every industrialized nation had its own atomic physicists; the nuclear age was on its way no matter what the United States decided.

Of course, no one knew for sure if, when the gadget was dropped from a B-29, it would detonate. It had to be tested. Furthermore, no bombs could be wasted. Only three existed—one in the form of a static apparatus to be exploded in the desert, and two as the real thing, dubbed "The Thin Man" and "The Fat Man" (by the time they became weapons of war, they would be renamed "Little Boy" and "Fat Man").

If Truman vetoed the use of the bomb, the military was ready to begin preparations for the invasion of Japan at once.

On Friday, July 13, exactly three months after Franklin Roosevelt's death, a truck delivered the detonator for the gadget by a secret road to a stretch of semidesert fifty miles from Alamogordo, New Mexico. A hundred-foot frame of iron scaffolding had been built against an old farmhouse, inside of which, at the last minute, the bomb core would be placed.

Before dawn on July 16, two B-29s took to the sky to radio in weather conditions. Ten miles away, the physicists on the project hunkered down in forts of reinforced concrete. When lightning flashes lit up the dark sky, the test was called off. But at 5:29 the impending sunrise was turning the sky to a light, calm gray. The bomb core was in place. A University of California physicist flipped a switch to activate a transmitter that then set off two other transmitters. Prearranged electrons moved into position.

No one saw the first flash. The atomic fire was beyond the scope of the human eye. A second later, all the physicists were jarred by the earth's vibration. A dazzling reflection appeared on hills far away. Hurricane-force winds swept across the desert with a deafening roar. The physicists grabbed anything they could find to stay upright. Stunned, excited, even shocked at what their science had created, they watched giant columns of clouds shoot into the dawn sky.

The smoke rose, and as the bomb's clouds climbed higher than Mount Everest, no one could stay silent. Their comments came: "Sunrise such as the world had never seen." "The sun can't hold a candle to it." One senior officer, less poetic, shouted, "I believe those long-haired boys have lost control."

Oppenheimer, the lead physicist, thought, "If the radiance of a thousand suns were to burst into the sky that would be like the splendor of the Mighty One. I am become Death, the shatterer of worlds."

By five-thirty the temperature at the bomb site was ten thousand times the temperature on the surface of the sun. In New Mexico and western Texas sleeping Americans were awakened by a mysterious storm.

A military general at the test site, witnessing the explosion, calmly said, "The war's over. One or two of those things and Japan will be finished."

And, of course, it was. The war that had killed more than sixty million, three percent of the world's population, was finally ended. All the world was changed, even medicine. When survivors of the blasts at Hiroshima and Nagasaki were found to have suppressed immune systems from nuclear radiation, the possibility of using X-ray beams to prepare a body to accept a foreign organ seemed reasonable. Eager to add to the science that Peter displayed in manipulating the immune system, Joe and Franny would eventually embrace the idea to follow whole-body irradiation with bone marrow transfusions to deactivate rejection, so as to create a welcoming host for a transplanted organ. Ironically, the idea—and funding— would come about as nations after World War II rushed to find treatments for survivors of nuclear war.

10

"You Were No Raving Beauty the First Time I Saw You, Either"

A LITTLE MORE than two years after Charles arrived at Valley Forge Hospital, in March 1946, he walked out for the first time. It would only be for the day, but the morning was set aside to see his son, now three years old. He had not seen Freddie since he was born, and Charles knew that his son would be scared out of his mind when he saw this man bandaged like a mummy and was told, *this is your dad.*

Most of Charles's face was swathed in bandages, the tip of them visible under his officer's cap. His neck was also covered with bandages, and he still wore big boxing gloves on his hands with his uniform's sleeves slit to fit around them.

This was also the first time he would be seen in public.

An icy wind blew. The ground was covered with snow. Miriam helped him step gingerly over an icy patch. Then she drove them to the apartment in Phoenixville where she and Freddie were living.

Charles put his arm around her and stared out the window, savoring the view of rolling hills flaked with snow. After so many months with his eyes covered, he wanted to study every line, every curve, every texture around him. Under his bandages, with his eyes closed, memories of the crash would often flash in his mind. He remembered sitting on the ground in Kurmitola while the flames lit up the sky. He would again see the smoke on his flight suit as he burned. Now with his eyes released from bandages, he could concentrate on the world outside of his mind.

Even with no ears, crippled hands, a rebuilt nose, and a "patchwork" face, he considered himself lucky just to be alive. Breathing in the invigorating air, he tested his homemade nose. In a few months he would be allowed to go home to Alabama. How good *that* would feel!—especially to reclaim the life that he and Miriam had planned—or rather, to begin the life he would now have to plan for himself.

Without hands to work with, he would have to find some way to make a living with his mind. All options were open, but he would not discuss any of them with anyone—not even with Miriam.

More reconstructive surgery was planned to put the final touches on his new face and especially his hands. He needed hands—he couldn't carry anything or even take money out of his billfold. Having functional hands seemed a priority. The plan was to release him soon from the hospital to live in the Phoenixville apartment with Miriam and Freddie while a few more surgeries were done, and also for all his skin grafts to fully heal.

For nearly two years, he had lived in the hospital, and during those years the world was being rearranged. America was not the country he had left at the beginning of the war. He would have to find a way to fit in.

While Miriam parked the car at the apartment house, Charles stood on the sidewalk. There was a group of small children carrying books on their way home from school. They stopped in front of him and stared. He could imagine what they were seeing: a man in a uniform with most of his face built of scars swathed in bandages. And with big boxing gloves on his hands. To them, he would seem like a monster—like something in a horror movie, or in a nightmare that had broken their sleep.

A little girl came closer. "Hi," she said. She ran back to join her group. She didn't seem frightened, just eager to rejoin her friends. She'd seemed only to want to take a closer look at him—not out of fear, but out of curiosity. Charles figured that since she lived near the Valley Forge Hospital, she was used to seeing soldiers in all sorts of frightening conditions. Probably she had become dull to the sights of someone like him. However, meeting his son, now aged three, could be a different matter.

He followed Miriam into the apartment where she and Freddie were living. Abruptly, the babysitter stood up. "I've got to run now," she blurted. Clearly startled at the sight of him, she threw her coat over her shoulders and raced from the house.

Charles laughed. "I hope that doesn't happen every time I meet somebody. The poor woman was scared half to death. I bet she's still running."

Miriam, instead of rattled, was relieved and encouraged by his sense of humor. "I'll never be afraid of how you handle people again," she added.

Now Freddie ran into the room. When he saw his father, he clamped his hands over his eyes. This was the reaction that Charles had dreaded. He would somehow have to find a way to become a father to a son who was deathly afraid of him.

Remembering the night his son had been born, when he had visited Miriam in the hospital and seen the prune-faced newborn lying by her side, Charles now quickly said, "That's all right, son. You were no raving beauty the first time I saw you, either."

Charles moved into the little apartment with Miriam and Freddie and went back weekly to the hospital for small repairs to his face and hands. In the months that followed, he and Miriam, with Freddie in the back seat, took drives, exploring the Pennsylvania countryside, enjoying each other. On these outings, they'd often stop for something to eat or to read a roadside marker that told of a Revolutionary War battle. As people stared at him, he learned to ease the embarrassing moment by calling out in his Alabama accent, "How y'all doing?" Usually, they called back too loudly, "Fine, fine," covering up their lack of composure.

To make friends with his son, Charles turned their small apartment living room into a wrestling arena. As Charles rolled on the floor with Freddie, growling and feigning attacks, his face and hands no longer mattered. To Freddie, his father became the best playmate he could ever have.

During one wrestling match, Charles's bandaged right eye was hit accidentally, and he instinctively knew he was in trouble. Miriam rushed him to the emergency room at Valley Forge.

The eye was fragile anyway. In one of his early surgeries, the scalpel had slipped and cut Charles's right eye so badly most of his vision was gone. Now, fear of infection in the injured eye was paramount. While that night he did not lose it, eventually he would. At the time, though, what he most cared about was getting back to Freddie for more wrestling matches.

He decided their apartment was too small. A new baby was on the way. Besides, more wrestling room was needed. They bought a modest house a mile from the Valley Forge Hospital.

Slowly, Charles's strength returned. The gauze bandages on his neck came off in stages, and he dreamed of returning to Alabama. In spring, he longed for the place where he had grown up. He wanted to see the farmers following their mules in the peanut and cotton fields again. He wanted to see the southern seasons move gently from fall to winter and spring to summer like a song changing keys.

In spring of 1947, he was promoted to major. The new baby came. They named him Andrew Michael, after one of the doctors at the hospital. Charles was told that he would have to wear his boxing gloves to protect his hands for two more years. Some of the skin grafts had not taken and had to be redone. By then, he'd been to the operating room sixty-five times. Finally, almost four years after the crash in India, he was told he could move to Alabama—as long as he came back at times for further surgery on his hands.

Miriam bought a bigger car. With all four of them packed into it, they headed to Alabama. Apprehension at going to where he would look like a stranger gnawed at him again. He would be the kind of stranger that no one had ever seen. In little Phoenixville, people had gotten used to him. Now he would have to enter a whole new place as who he had become, even though it would be the place where he had grown up. Would they, like Miriam, faint when they first saw him?

He reminded himself that when Miriam had seen him for the first time it was before the months of plastic surgery that gave him a mask to wear out into the world. Often now he studied himself in the mirror. At least the different colors of the skin that had been taken from his arms, legs, hips, and stomach seemed to come together in one color. His uniform's cap covered the red flaps of harvested skin on his head, which of course could never grow hair. His nose was still being shaped, which, along with his right eye, was covered. He told himself that the black patch over his injured eye would be the focus of most people's stares.

As Miriam drove, she planned their long trip to Alabama, thinking of Freddie and Andy in the back seat. "We'll stop for the night and leave early in the morning."

"That's fine," he said. "Just take it easy driving. I want to get home in one piece."

The irony of what he had just said hit them both. They laughed and then laughed with another sort of relieved joy when they turned onto the road to their hometown.

Settling in a rented house near Dothan, where he had grown up, Charles first went to see his family. His adoptive father looked at him and said, "You look fine," as if Charles were the same man who had gone to India four years earlier. His aunt added, "But you could use a little weight," and rattled off what she had cooked for supper that night: country ham, corn bread, grits . . .

With no hands—or what was left of them, and still encased in boxing gloves to protect the fragile skin grafts and healing bones—what could he do? He couldn't be a mechanic. He couldn't be a farmer. He couldn't work machinery. He couldn't even take money out of his wallet. Or carry anything—not even his two sons.

Those who knew him in his little hometown began to give advice: raise turkeys. Raise chickens. He could collect his government pension. He could take it easy. He could just sit back and enjoy life.

Turkeys? Chickens? Pension? There was other advice. Sit in a recliner, listen to the radio, or maybe look at one of those new-fangled things that looked like a Bendix washing machine with a little circular screen that showed pictures. The thing called a television? Not likely. Besides, that thing seemed too strange to put in a living room.

He said to Miriam, "God didn't give me back my life so that I could waste it away sitting back and collecting a pension." He made it clear that he had not fought so hard to stay alive to whittle away the rest of his days, relaxing.

Finding a way to make a living by using his mind was what he needed.

Like many soldiers returning from the war, he felt not only the optimism of a new world order for young families, but an obligation and desire to replace the lives that had been lost. Having many children was his and Miriam's hope. The American dream of owning a house, a car, and having many children to help replace the friends killed in the war was contagious.

Miriam was inside feeding the new baby when she heard the honking of a horn outside. That blaring horn meant Charles was in a hurry or had some important news. She rushed out to the driveway of their new Alabama home with Andy in her arms and Freddie close behind. There was Charles in a new truck. Freddie jumped on the running board and looked in at his dad who did not look like any dad anywhere, ever.

"Where did you get that?" Miriam asked.

"I just bought it. Ain't it a beauty? It's our first investment."

What in the world was he talking about, she wanted to know, to which he boldly announced, "We're in the construction business. I bought the truck and a lot to build a house on. Now I'm going out to hunt me some people who know how to build houses."

"Do you have money left to do that?"

"A little from my military pay. I bought the truck and then I mortgaged it to the bank for the money to buy the lot."

Miriam walked to the side of the truck. She looked in and smiled at him. He was dressed in a khaki shirt, jeans, and a hunting cap. With the same determination he used in Flying the Hump day after day, he was setting out to make his way in the life he had fought so hard to save.

11

"So I Can't Be Too Bad"

By 1947, Peter's magical mix of traits was becoming known. He was so precise in designing his experiments and carrying them out that other scientists immediately wanted to duplicate them. The Nobel Prize-winning chemist Sir Norman Haworth, at the University of Birmingham in England, took notice and invited Peter to interview for a position as professor in the zoology department. There Peter sat, the interview committee staring at him, while Sir Norman handed him a test tube of a white crystalline powder he said was type H pneumococcal polysaccharide and commanded, "Discuss!"

Nothing in Peter's study of zoology had prepared him for this, but at least he knew the form of pneumonia in the test tube. True to his restless curiosity, he had studied on his own the dramatic reactions of the mild form of the bacteria when it transformed into the one that almost invariably killed a patient. With his usual flair and passion, he began discussing the dangers of the test tube powder to living organisms to the point of boring the interview committee into fidgeting, while also dazzling them with his wide-ranging intellect. Immediately, they offered him the chair of zoology. At only thirty-two he now became known not only as zoologist Peter Medawar but also as the "boy professor."

In Birmingham, Jean found a lovely eighteenth-century house for them, surrounded by an acre of garden. At this time, she was heavily involved in caring for her and Peter's family of four children: two boys, two girls. With the help of two au pairs, she ran the household, cooked meals, nursed childhood illnesses, kept the coal stove filled and tended, and eventually estimated the likely distance of cloth diapers she had washed and dried on an outside clothesline, should they be pinned end-to-end in a straight line over the years. At least five miles worth, she figured. It was also at this time that Peter took off his student clothes of jeans and a pullover and began wearing a dark gray suit with a white shirt—every day. For the rest of his life, he never deviated from his daily gray suit.

———————

THAT SAME YEAR, Joe was released from the army, and, as he made plans to return to Boston, he carried with him the experience of caring for Charles. He marveled at how all those who met Charles saw that a will to live could overcome enormous odds. No science could explain Charles's nearly miraculous survival. Eventually, there would be greater understanding of the body's response to injury and the role of the immune system. In time, Joe would surmise that the weakness of Charles's body likely prevented his immune system from quickly attacking the cadaver's borrowed skin, allowing the skin grafts to last longer than was ever expected. But the spiritual side of Charles's determination to live could never be measured, nor could it have been predicted. A patient's will to live would forever remain a secret, unique to each.

Much to Joe's delight, he was accepted back to complete his surgical residency at the Peter Bent Brigham in Boston. He was especially pleased to find Franny on the staff as an instructor in surgery. Not yet the giant he would become, Franny was still notable from his role in the Cocoanut Grove nightclub fire. To wet-behind-the-ears interns and residents under him, he was scary.

When Franny walked into a room, the atmosphere changed. When he walked down a hall, his presence could always be felt. Some called it the bearing of raw power, as if an eagle or lion were nearby, watching. But at the same time, he was always paternal, quick to rescue a colleague who was stumbling. Or hesitating. And he was only thirty-four.

When he appeared, people wanted to follow—unless they suffered from the all-too-common trait of envy and made a quick, sharp criticism of Franny. Words like *arrogant* and even *vindictive* were heard at times. As with anyone on a high-octane pursuit of excellence, he could leave collateral damage in his wake. On his battlefield against illness, everyone was drafted and required to fight. His favorite saying was from Ecclesiastes 7:35: "Be not slow to visit the sick . . . "

During the war years, the Brigham had become a hub of innovation. Knowing what crush syndrome had revealed about the resilience of the kidneys, the hospital established a program to explore innovative treatments for renal failure. The year 1947, so significant to Joe, Peter, and Franny, was also the year that Willem Kolff emigrated to the United States and visited the Brigham. He fascinated the staff, telling them how he devised a dialysis machine. Even though he had no machine with him, he left a blueprint. And Franny noted that the Brigham renal team "quickly improved [Kolff's invention] into a usable washing device to remove toxins from the blood of those patients whose kidneys were off duty either temporarily or permanently." They now used polyethylene tubing instead of sausage casing and a rotation apparatus to filter the blood. With a dialysis machine in place to keep patients alive temporarily, the

Brigham's commitment to renal research and innovation grew more solid.

What Joe had learned at Valley Forge in general and plastic surgery, coupled with his witness of Charles's long-lasting allografts, encouraged him to explore his seemingly off-the-wall idea of transplantation. A laboratory at the Brigham was already doing experimental transplants, using dogs as research models. The veins and arteries of a dog were close enough in size to those of a human to make the research feasible. But Joe was only a resident with years of training still ahead.

At least he was no longer called a "pup," the nickname for an intern. And he was quietly waiting to see if his farfetched idea of "spare-parts" surgery could indeed give those dying of kidney failure a second life.

Many in the traditional medical profession thought organ transplantation was so out of the mainstream that the idea of it was best left to basic scientists to solve, not surgeons. Whenever Joe commented on the value of the program, he was often warned, "Joe, don't get involved in that. It will never work, and you may ruin your whole future." Research fellows who considered joining the effort were often told that the surgeons working on transplantation were "a bunch of fools."

Joe was not one to argue. Few knew of the deep stubbornness hidden under his cheerful disposition and easygoing manner. Not many would guess that lurking within was as much grit as Franny showed, and a tenacious curiosity that, once awakened, would fuel his ferocious work ethic.

Soon, the Brigham's reputation for treating renal disease spread. On any given day in Boston, patients could be seen arriving at the Brigham with a yellow tint to their skins. Physicians across the country began referring their patients as a last hope. All were young; all were suffering from one of the three diseases to cause kidney failure.

For centuries these illnesses became known to the lay public through characters in novels, or by way of the pages of history. Bright's disease, also known as glomerulonephritis—meaning the inflammation of the kidney involving the little cups (glomeruli) that filter the blood—was first identified in 1836 when London physician Richard Bright described *uremia* as the condition arriving from waste products collecting in the blood from failing kidneys. The second cause, chronic pyelonephritis (nephritis), begins in the kidney drainage system in the pelvis. The third common disease is the malformation of the organs themselves with cysts in the kidneys or else fused or joined abnormally, known as "horseshoe kidney."

In older people, hardening of the arteries produces the majority of kidney failure, but in all, the outward signs are the same: pale skin with a yellow-pasty look, loss of appetite, loss of weight, and the inability to excrete water and salt properly, which produces swollen ankles. Fluid collects in the abdomen, which in Dickens's novels was often described as a character having "dropsy." As fictional characters and real people died from kidney disease, the public began to know at least the symptoms.

Theodore Roosevelt's young wife, Alice Lee, died of Bright's disease as a complication of childbirth. (Her daughter and namesake, Alice Longworth, years later would captivate the nation with her mischief, leading President Theodore Roosevelt to say, "I can either run the nation or I can attend to Alice, but I cannot possibly do both.") American history was again marked by Bright's disease when President Woodrow Wilson's beloved wife, Ellen, died in the White House of the dreaded illness.

The result of the diseases often brought suffering to all as the victims died slowly and agonizingly. Watching such a death frequently traumatized family members, putting strains on their emotional health. The call to save the young, dying of kidney disease, never grew silent.

———

JOE AND FRANNY were men who made sense of the world by what they learned in their years in medical school. With Franny entering Harvard Medical School in 1935 and Joe in 1940, their medical educations were essentially the same. It was their backgrounds that marked them as different. Franny, as the son of privilege, and Joe, as the grandson of immigrants, said everything about what the idea of America intended. That they would end up being in the same revered medical school only years apart equipped them to practice medicine with the same skill. Yet, at that time, the practice of medicine was as much an art as a science, and they learned to be doctors at a time when few diagnostic tools existed.

They relied on what their eyes could observe, what they could hear through a stethoscope, what their hands could feel, and what their hearts could interpret as being left unspoken. In that way, they were men whose experiences of youth would last throughout their long lifetimes, as well as color their visions to leave a mark on medicine that would be timeless.

Joe grew up in an idyllic moment in America. Lindbergh had just made the first trans-Atlantic flight. Flying was so new that when Joe was ten years old he would look up whenever he heard a plane crawling across the sky. Everyone did. With Franklin Delano Roosevelt's election in 1932, a feeling of security spread across the nation. No one thought much about Hitler and Mussolini. They were just two comical overseas dictators with no real importance to Americans. In Milford, Massachusetts, where Joe was growing up, he, along with all American children, was coming of age without fear and with visions of prosperous, happy futures.

Often Joe would walk alone to the town park in Milford to look for a pick-up game of baseball. In spring, he studied the leaves dappling the sidewalk. In winter, he walked to Louisa Lake or Hopedale Pond for a pick-up game of hockey. Listening to the sound of his boots crunching the snow seemed nature's way of making music. And since he was born on April Fool's Day, 1919, he felt he'd been given a seasonless canvas on which to mount his playful sense of humor.

Even as a boy, he displayed one trait above all others—the ability to think beyond himself, not a trait generally helpful in the pursuit of survival. Where and how he acquired it is as spellbinding as the innate dexterity that led to his becoming a skilled surgeon. As a child, Joe was also compassionate beyond the usual.

Passio, meaning *suffering,* and *com,* meaning *with,* is the only common value shared among Buddhists, Confucians, Taoists, and Christians. Some philosophers argue that the ability to feel goodwill for a fellow life traveler must be taught. Perhaps the best and simplest comment on compassion is the one Leonardo da Vinci made when he advised that "as a well-spent day brings happy sleep, so a life well spent brings happy death." And that would certainly prove to be true for Joe.

If indeed Joe was born with an unusual slice of compassion, models in his family strengthened his concern for others, beginning with his immigrant grandparents. They infected him with their dreams. They insisted that he get the best education America offered. Taking their advice, Joe stuffed his bookshelf with titles that gave him his first heroes, books whose pages he read so often they eventually slipped from their spines: *Arrowsmith, Microbe Hunters, An American Doctor's Odyssey,* and especially *Memoirs of a Small-town Surgeon,* by John Brooks Wheeler. This last one gave him a first glimpse of the marble quadrangle of Harvard Medical School, which also quietly teased him with the thought: *Might I aim for that school, too?* Whenever someone asked him as a young boy what he wanted to be when he grew up, Joe's answer always was "a surgeon." His family doctor, who compassionately treated his family's everyday illnesses, became a beloved ideal.

Listening to his father regret that he had not been able to afford college, but instead had gone straight from high school to law school, Joe knew that a traditional education was highly prized. So he worked hard. Watching his father voraciously read the classics—devouring novels, mythology, Greek and Roman histories and biographies by the score—also convinced him that a liberal education was to be cherished. In high school Joe learned how to be organized, to pay attention to detail, to practice self-discipline, to hone his natural stubbornness until he would pick up a problem and shake it silly, either solving it or leaving it better off than when he found it. Even though his father eventually became a judge, a volunteer to help immigrants obtain citizenship, and an advisor to help immigrants get credit from local banks, his wistful yearning for the confidence of those with established credentials left an impression on Joe. His father never stopped reminding him to get the best education he could. Later, as a comfort to his father, Joe liked to point out the accomplishments of Harry Truman, who also compensated for his lack of a college education.

Joe's mother often recited her parents' story, with pride in its grit—of how, at the ages of nineteen and seventeen, they left

Italy, boarded a ship headed to America with name tags around their necks, and traveled twenty-nine days sharing close quarters with cattle, to settle in Rhode Island. Joe watched his mother always speaking Italian with her own mother—dressed in black with her old-world ways—during family visits to ease her mother's discomfort of being in a country whose language would always be foreign to her.

In time, Joe's mother became the first woman of Italian heritage to teach in the Massachusetts public school system. Loving politics, she was honored by a special resolution in the Massachusetts legislature for her contributions to the commonwealth. But it was *her* father who gave Joe the story he relished telling. It was this Italian grandfather who was a juggler of ideas. He ran a sand and gravel business, was a successful undertaker, an insurance salesman, and also the owner and operator of a soft drink processing plant on the first floor of their home while renting out the third floor to another family.

For hours, Joe stood beside his grandfather's drink machine, which sent bottles of orangeade rattling on an automated journey to be filled and capped. Since Joe was allowed to grab as many bottles of the orange pop as he wanted, he loved saying that, early on, he realized the value of having kidneys that work.

On Sunday evenings, Joe's father would invite him into his study where they read and discussed the classics. On the day Joe graduated from high school, his father presented him with Marshall's four-volume biography of George Washington, which Joe would always keep with him, moving it from place to place.

His self-discipline and work ethic paid off. As he was about to graduate from Milford High School as an all-around athlete and salutatorian, he applied to Holy Cross College. In his interview there, when asked why he had chosen Holy Cross rather than Dartmouth or Harvard, where he had also been accepted, Joe said he wanted a strong liberal arts education. His interviewer nodded his approval. And that's when Joe gave loose rein to his love for literature, music, and memorizing poetry. He knew medical school would be heavily weighted with sciences so he valued his time with these other subjects. Despite the hard work and long hours of study, he stayed true to his temperament; no one day was less wonderful than the next. And in 1940, when he graduated with honors from Holy Cross, he was admitted to Harvard Medical School a week later.

Now that he was on the path of his hero John Brooks Wheeler, he made a note to himself: *I've been thinking about my future. At first, I never thought I'd be successful. I had doubts about getting admitted to medical school—always figured so many fellows round here were so much better than I. But they were rejected and I was accepted. So I can't be too bad.*

During his first year in medical school, he gave barely a nod toward the thought that he would be anything other than "a good doctor" like his family's beloved Dr. Curley. But one day in his second year, when he was in the lab of his pathology instructor, the professor slipped a few of his slides from his study on inflammation under the microscope's lens for Joe to have a look. As Joe bent over to see the slide, he watched cells accumulate in one site but not in another. Excitement filled him, instantly. It was a moment he never wanted to let go of.

Later, when working on a paper to present to the Boylston Medical Society, he realized he was about to head in a direction that he never would have predicted. He jotted down a note to himself: *I want to, some day, read up on old surgical operations for ideas which, although impractical then, now will be useful in conjunction with chemotherapy, a new concept, and other developments. There are so many ideas in them and so much to learn about that the days are too short.*

Eventually, he would say, "Naively, I had thought that medicine would be taught as a trade with a dash of humanity thrown in. And while I knew that research was a fundamental part of that trade, I did not expect it to be an important part of my medical career. Frankly, I was worried about being smart enough to graduate."

———————

WHEN FRANNY ENTERED in 1935, he discovered he couldn't even brag about getting accepted to Harvard. During the Depression, few could afford the school, which accepted everyone. Furthermore, Harvard Medical School was a simple graduate school. No government funding. No corporate funding. Tuition was four hundred dollars.

The science was solid but nothing to write home about. With a two-tiered hospital system for teaching, there were charity wards and private wings. For most of its existence, the medical school had been nothing more than a diploma factory until it was dramatically changed by Harvard president Charles Eliot, who, in 1870, introduced entrance examinations and measures of achievement for students before they could be awarded their MD degree. No malpractice suits, no open-ended government payment systems requiring excessive billing, no paperwork by insurance companies telling physicians what to do—furthermore, a doctor never had to know how to type. Instead, students learned to talk into a Dictaphone, to enunciate clearly, to get rid of any accent, to get the work done by unraveling case histories and treatment plans unendingly for hundreds and hundreds of patients, while a transcriptionist, usually a woman hidden in the bowels of the hospital, typed it up.

In Franny's class of 120 students, his studies were serene, with little hard science—an education still being criticized, in spite of Eliot's long-ago reforms, for being a factory churning out diplomas with, it seemed, more of a commitment to community service than to the achievement of learning. The student body was homogenous and limited. It was after World War II that medical practice and training changed.

In 1945, Harvard Medical School's teaching hospitals contained charity beds, reserved for the state's patients. Many patients were cared for as a charitable service by the physicians who came from their private practices, receiving no pay for treating charity patients. They came for the prestige of the academic appointment and the privilege of teaching. Actually, they were hoping for the possibility to be appointed to the staff. Interns and residents' salaries were about twenty-five dollars a month, or sometimes nothing at all.

There Franny was—settling into his first classes, studying anatomy, physiology, and biochemistry, dissecting his first cadaver, taking home a box of bones to study, discovering the beauty and efficiency of the human body, and learning that, for the sake of sanity, death had to be compartmentalized. Hospital double-talk protected medical students from the reality of failure. Patients who died were referred to as being "transferred to ward X" or "sent to Allen Street," which was the name of the road behind Mass General where the hearses came.

Remaining disconnected was essential; otherwise students dropped out or headed to a field other than clinical medicine. Early on, a student's capacity for connection to his own humanity was displayed while examining his first patient. Whether a student showed empathy or coldness or had an interest in the disease only from a scientific viewpoint was now revealed. Some students came to empathy naturally, others slowly. Some never connected with their shared humanity. Through his imagination, rather than experience, Franny could readily understand what it must feel like to be ripped from an everyday life, to be the captive of an illness that a patient was helpless to defeat, alone.

In the midst of his second and third year of clinical study, in keeping with the school's requirement, he delivered twelve babies in patients' homes, traveling to an assigned, and impoverished, area of Boston. There, in poor homes without anesthesia, with instruments sterilized by boiling on a gas stove (as long as the gas company had not turned it off), and with perhaps a single dangling electric bulb, he brought his required number of babies into the world. Sometimes the husband would be in the home drunk, and sometimes there were bug-eyed children huddled in another room. If the labor became troubled, Franny was taught to give the husband a nickel to go to a pay phone to call for an intern to drive over to help. Often the mother herself would instruct, "Now you tie the cord and cut it."

In those first years of his medical studies, Franny was drawn to making a patient well, quickly. He began thinking of becoming a surgeon. During the previous fifty years, surgery had been monumentally improved, beginning with the publication of Lister's landmark paper in 1867 on the necessity of surgical cleanliness. Before then, surgeons operated in street clothes, never cleaned their instruments between patients, and never suspected that they themselves might be the sources for spreading infection. The concept of germs opened the pathway for understanding bacteria and infection, and the discovery of anesthesia with ether—introduced through the practice of dentistry—changed everything. These innovations, along with a full understanding of how to set broken bones, moved surgery into a new age. Previously, limbs with broken bones had been amputated. The chest was never entered, the abdomen, rarely. But, over time, surgery did become a way to make patients well, quickly.

As a field of specialization, surgery took on requirements of its own. The dedication became daunting. The going theory was that medical students, and especially surgical interns, should not be married, a custom promoted mainly by the famous surgeon Harvey Cushing, who was engaged to his future wife for more than six years before finally booking their wedding.

For Franny it was different. He had fallen so deeply and forever in love with Laurie at the age of fifteen that when he graduated from Harvard—and she, from Sarah Lawrence—they went to their parents and announced they wanted to get married. No one was surprised. In 1935, Franny had only one goal in mind: to enter medical school with Laurie by his side.

They married on June 24 at the Congregational Church in Winnetka, Illinois, and immediately took off in a Ford Model A sedan with attached tin cans rattling on the pavement. They headed to Milwaukee for their wedding night. But on the way, they were overtaken by a sudden, frightening lightning storm. Sparks flew from the electric power lines. The downpour pelted so hard on the metal roof of the car, nothing else could be heard. The deluge was so torrential that Franny pulled to the side of the road. From there, he and Laurie watched nature's energy rain down on the flat, hot plains. In moments, it was all over, followed by a spectacular sunset. But the experience would remain in Franny's mind to eventually haunt him fifty years later when he would look back on it as a foreshadowing for the day he would be parted from Laurie.

By the time he stepped into the anatomy lab at medical school, they were settled as newlyweds in an apartment near the school. As one of only two married medical students, he was set apart from the others. But Franny didn't care. Being married to Laurie was even more glorious than he had imagined.

After his first week of the anatomy course, he took his assigned box of bones home to study. He kept them under the bed and, being a perfectionist, pulled them out to study so often that Laurie reminded him, "Alright, Moorie, let's take the bones back to the morgue." But it was not just his type-A personality driving him to be a perfect student; he was also unsettled by what he was facing. The first day he walked into the anatomy lab, paired with four other classmates to dissect a cadaver, he had never before seen a dead person.

The body on which he was to learn the awe-inspiring systems that make up a human held little resemblance to the real beauty of a living being. Brown, dried out, smelling of formaldehyde, the flesh was stiff and cold. With a scalpel and forceps, he gingerly exposed and sometimes clumsily revealed the inner workings of the biology that once had walked, talked, had thoughts and dreams. The questions began coming: how did that person die? How did he live? The cadaver next to his with classmates huddled over it had a bullet lodged in the heart. But Franny found no bullet or obvious cause of death in the cadaver he spent so much time exploring.

Looking at the brain, he believed that, despite its complexity, it was also a dwelling place. The thinking mind existed in a brain that converted energy into thought. When thought ceased, the essence of a person no longer lived there, though the physical brain remained.

He was struck with the mind-body dualism. All of his classmates were. They shared questions that had challenged the most profound philosophers for centuries. Franny had always interpreted the soul as an "epiphenomenon of the mind that requires an observed, a 'third party' for its validation and to achieve reality." He thought of the mind as an expansion of the brain and the soul as an extension and an expression of that mind. This philosophy became part of his emerging picture of the former person that now was the lifeless body on which he cut and took apart while learning to be a physician.

Eventually it became clear: his job would be to keep the dwelling place for the soul suitable for habitation. The anatomy instructor, knowing that each class awoke to the same questions, taught them not to say, "I am a body, I have soul," but rather, "I am a soul, I live in a body." The study of human anatomy then became settled where the students could manage it.

Anatomy was put where it belonged: as the structure to serve as a dwelling place. In time, Franny realized that "injury and disease can so destroy that warm dwelling place that it is no longer habitable, and the dweller—energy, mind, and soul—had best be permitted to depart." In those circumstances, he would have to learn to let life go.

Exposure to these new thoughts of human existence was exciting and exhausting. Instead of feeling overwhelmed and eternally confused, he found it thrilling. When he was introduced to his first patients and taught the methods of examination and differential diagnosis, he saw that some of his classmates found dealing with patients to be stressful, with no ability to connect, to care, to imagine the ravages of disease on the emotions. In the anatomy lab, they had already learned to be disconnected to some degree. As Franny entered his surgical training, he realized he would be even closer to the reality of life and death and needed to "develop skin of exactly the right thickness," so as not to be crippled by overwhelming emotion.

He saw that if a surgeon's skin was too thin, he was whipped by death, brooding, and worrying, was unable to sleep, and would become cut off from learning new ideas. By watching his classmates, he learned that the middle ground of sensitivity was either inborn or acquired from one's parents, probably in childhood. While he thought that compassion and empathy could not be learned, it could be strengthened by example, and he vowed to become one of those surgeons and teachers who would model the necessary balance.

As a surgeon, treating patients became exhilarating to Franny. His intellectual curiosity naturally led him to want to delve into *why* and *how* the body responded to surgery. Already he was mapping a course to become one of those surgeon-scientists in the vein of Harvey Cushing. He was intrigued by what he called "the chemistry of getting well."

On the night in his fourth year of medical school when he was offered a residency in surgery at the nine Harvard teaching hospitals, he joined his classmates in a rowdy celebration. He drank too much, and Laurie propped him up against a wall. Later, she stuffed him into the car for the drive home. The next day, he was back at work, nursing a hangover, rushing from room to room tending to patients' needs, and in awe that Laurie had somehow managed to take care of his sorry self. Soon, her duties at home were all-consuming, too. She gave birth to their first daughter. In time, four more children would follow.

To take a break from being on the biology battleground, the resident group became partners in pranks, often led by Franny, especially in tricking their professors. When he noticed in the surgeons' lounge that photographs of former staff hung on the walls, going back even to the physicians in the early days soon after photography was invented, he egged on his own resident group to dress up like them and have their picture taken. There they were: looking out of their modern photo frame wearing black frock coats, mustaches, beards, and expressions as if nursing green-apple stomachaches. Their piercing eyes could bore a hole into any young intern. It took several months for the phony photo to be discovered. But it remained there long enough to enjoy the sight of a bunch of young whippersnappers trying to look like old Boston Brahmins in the days of the discovery of anesthesia and sawed-off limbs.

If these hijinks relieved the seriousness of the biology battle, they could not relieve the sorrow and distress of failures. Franny considered the first death of one of his patients to be his fault, and he would never forget it. Ten days after he had operated to remove a cancerous tumor in his patient's breast, she got up to walk to the bathroom and fell to the floor, dead. At that time, patients stayed in bed ten days to two weeks after such surgery.

Distraught, Franny went to her husband to tell him and openly stated that he thought her death was his fault. An autopsy showed that a massive clot deep in the vein of her leg had traveled snakelike to her lung, which during those years prior to the forties was not recognized as a threat. Franny continued to chide himself, thinking that if he had been a little more sensitive the day before to a rise in her temperature and pulse, he might have suspected that clot. Eventually, with enough of these sudden deaths, procedures were changed. It became normal practice to get patients up and walking after surgery to prevent pulmonary embolisms.

As much as he wanted to outwit nature's unpredictable complications, there were limits to what he could do. Restricted by the unknown, bound by what medicine had yet to discover, he had to endure one of the most haunting deaths that enveloped the whole surgical team. It was the case of an infant boy, born with the fairly common condition of pyloric stenosis, in which an overgrowth of muscle narrows the outlet for the stomach so that the baby has severe and repeated vomiting. Franny performed the operation in textbook form.

He had worked many times with the nurse giving the anesthesia, and he trusted her completely. While he was writing the orders to be given back in the child's hospital room, she lovingly picked up the unconscious baby to carry him back to his ward. In those days, there were no postoperative recovery rooms or intensive care units. The nurse walked down the hall to the infant's ward with the baby's head draped on her shoulder. By the time Franny changed his clothes from his surgical greens and went to the infants' ward, he found the baby lying ashen pale, dead. The animal-like wail of the mother's grief would never be completely wiped from his memory. If a moment in his life as a surgeon could be erased, it would be that one. It was the impetus for his lifelong study into the body's response to surgery, for the experience taught him how much was to be learned about surgery's effects on the body.

It took a while to figure out what had happened—that the deep anesthesia paralyzed the infant's blood vessel reflexes that kept the blood flowing against gravity, up from the legs and lower part of the body to the brain and heart. In an infant those reflexes are not yet strong. Later, Franny wrote, "When the anesthetist lovingly picked up the child and held him against her shoulder, she unwittingly restrained him in the upright posture." And in that position the stagnant blood pooled in his legs. The brain, robbed of blood, started to die and, with it, the drive for respiration. Death by crucifixion occurs in the same way: blood flows to the feet and legs with fainting soon followed by death.

Franny never spoke harshly to the anesthetist or blamed her. With the child's face against her shoulder, she couldn't study his face to see the effects of what was happening to him. Criticism and false reassurances were not necessary. Franny knew how the nurse felt. In response to the death, the practice of surgical procedures was changed. Laying infants down in a wheeled crib to be taken to the recovery room became standard practice.

During the six years of his surgical training, the days were as long as he wanted to make them. And he made them long indeed. Death from disease or injury was the constant war, and he loved being on the front lines.

As soon as he finished his residency, he was offered the position of instructor in surgery. He was not an ordinary type of young surgeon—that was clear from his exemplary performance during the Cocoanut Grove tragedy. And his commitment to researching burn care afterward established him as being the rare breed of surgeon-scientist.

From his intense study of burn victims, he took on a study of the body's normal fluid content, wanting to learn what the normal amount of water is in the body and how much is sodium and potassium. In general, what changes occur after injury or surgery? At that time, astonishingly, no one knew how to measure the amount of water in the human body. And treatment errors came from not knowing how much fluid there was to determine dehydration, loss of sodium, and the like. Franny set about studying the chemistry of getting well. No one before him had done this, not to the degree and dedication he brought to the science.

Since he had seen burned patients go into shock or die in the first twenty-four hours from inadequate fluid treatment, he now took it on as a research subject. He used techniques of nuclear physics and injected into a patient a carefully measured dose of heavy water, the nonradioactive isotope of hydrogen. When this water was mixed with the body's ordinary water, the dilution of the heavy water would show the body's total water volume. It sounded simple, but it wasn't. It took Franny two and half years to get the results that his meticulous standards required. But the result was that today, his early research led to the method that can give the readout on a patient in minutes.

His reputation for around-the-clock dedication to improving patient care became a story line for those training under him. After a duck-hunting trip, his residents had a grand time imitating him as he sat in a duck blind in the midst of winter, his rifle propped on his shoulder, a pencil in his fingers scratching madly on a pad to calculate the rate of body heat falling by the minute. When a colleague called over, "What'd you find out, Franny?" he crisply yelled back, "It is damn cold out here."

He never stopped. He spent so much time at the hospital that as a joke and a favor, his neighbor mowed MOORE in his overgrown lawn. The truth was, he was on a fast track to eminence, and he himself said, "I led a whirlwind existence including both research and practice, tolerable only to one of irrational ambition, unforgivable ego, and insufferable determination—possible only for one with a supportive wife who possessed an inexhaustible reservoir of forgiveness." That reservoir even included Laurie's getting into a wheelchair and letting Franny wheel her into grand rounds, where about a hundred students and physicians sat listening to the presentation of an illness and treatment. Only later did the audience find out that the fake patient was the lecturer's wife.

With the burgeoning activity in his research lab, he was named simultaneously to two of the most revered posts in American surgery: surgeon-in-chief at the Brigham Hospital and Moseley Professor of Surgery at Harvard Medical School. It was 1948. Franny was thirty-five. He would soon publish the thousand-plus-page volume of *The Metabolic Care of the Surgical Patient*, listing his chief lab technician, Margaret R. Ball, as coauthor. And soon, too, his colleagues would affectionately say as they saw him coming down the hall, "Here comes the Mose."

The Metabolic Care of the Surgical Patient was a medical landmark. Other landmark publications would follow, but already Franny was making a universal declaration that a surgeon's responsibility was to take care of the whole patient. He was now in a league with the most eminent American surgeons, a list led by Harvey Cushing, who held the Moseley Professorship of Surgery at the Brigham when its doors opened in 1913 and was the first surgeon to request that research laboratories be located in the medical school.

The Peter Bent Brigham was the gift of a successful Boston merchant who endowed the hospital from funds drawn from his accumulated wealth, which came partly from real estate and partly from his savvy investments. The hospital was built immediately adjacent to Harvard Medical School, with its mission to care for the sick poor of Suffolk County. Within twenty-five years of its opening, the Brigham was known worldwide as a premier hospital where excellence was a matter of course. Its reputation was largely based on the work of Harvey Cushing, who, with his emphasis on the science of medicine for more than twenty years, became the model for the surgeon-scientist, developing the field of neurosurgery and also creating a chart universally used to monitor the patient's course under anesthesia. The motivation for the chart came from his own despair when he himself as a young surgeon-in-training administered anesthesia that caused a patient's death. He rebelled against the tradition that a young surgeon could administer anesthesia for a minor procedure, therefore advancing the study of anesthesia by demanding that doctors specialize in the field.

When Franny was training Joe, just released from military duty, he was also training other young surgeons, many of whom came straight out of medical units near battle sites. War-hardened, technically advanced, sometimes even beyond the abilities of their professors, they were fearless. Not much could rattle them.

When a first-year resident accidentally cut the finger of an older resident during a surgery, sending blood flowing onto the table and onto their surgical greens, the older resident barked, "Here," holding up his finger after he stitched it up himself. "Now tie it," he commanded, dangling the thread for the younger surgeon to knot.

The war had done more than rearrange the world of nations. It had pushed medicine into being more than a four-year degree at a technical school. And now, the Brigham would become the forerunner in the seemingly off-the-wall idea of trying to transplant an organ.

Franny and Joe, in the tradition of American pioneers, would be among the first to take it on.

And the first to pull it off.

12

Doable

TWO MONTHS AFTER Charles was settled near his hometown of Dothan, Alabama, he got on a plane to fly back to Valley Forge for more reconstructive surgery on his hands. He went alone so that Miriam could stay in Dothan to watch over the construction of their new home.

Not until he got on the plane did he realize how much he'd come to depend on Miriam. When the flight attendant placed a tray of food in front of him, he was unable to hold the fork or spoon. Seeing his dilemma, she came back and fed him, and when the plane landed in Philadelphia, she said, "You'll need some help with your bag. I'll meet you at the baggage counter after we land." She carried his bag to the taxi stand outside the terminal. When he started to pay the cab driver, he realized he couldn't get his wallet out of his pocket. Holding out his bandaged hands, the cab driver nodded, saying, "It's all right. I'll get your wallet for you. Where is it?" When he tried to tip the driver, the driver waved the money away. "I should tip you," he said.

That night from the hospital, after a nurse fed Charles, spoon to mouth, as he helplessly had to let her, he called Miriam. The nurse also had to dial the phone for him and hold the receiver to his ear. The next day, after surgery, he fought the pain as he had before. Ten days later, he was ready to leave for home.

Again, the return trip held the same humiliations: someone reaching for his wallet to pay for a taxi, someone to carry his bag, someone to feed him. When Miriam met him at the airport in Birmingham, she sensed his mood, saying he was like a rattlesnake about to strike. "What's the matter, Charles?"

"You know what I'm waiting for?" he replied. "I'm waiting for the day when I can carry my own luggage and count my own money."

There were other trips to Valley Forge for more reconstructive surgery, but he refused to let Miriam accompany him. They had added more kids to the big family they planned, and, as Charles said, "Somebody has to watch over things when I'm not around." He was also watching over the family's financial future. In a few years, the first television set would appear in Dothan, a happening that would set off a refrain in Charles's mind like an old song. Those strange-looking contraptions resembling a washing machine that sat in the living room had to receive signals from somewhere. That *somewhere* might be a good investment to look into.

––––––

As a resident, Joe was expanding his surgical knowledge, following Franny's treatments in the aftercare of surgical patients. Franny even coached Joe on other skills, advising him not to be impatient or outspoken, to guard his tongue in the operating room and in conferences. Franny's advice was easy for Joe to take as it fit in with his even disposition and non-confrontational personality. Soon he realized that by not antagonizing the staff, he was rarely misinterpreted. Surgery required fine-tuned teamwork, and taking Franny's advice meant the days moved smoothly.

For three months, Joe worked across the street in neurosurgery at Boston Children's Hospital using his skill in plastic surgery gained at Valley Forge. He treated children's facial deformities that came either from birth or injury and found that giving these children new faces to wear out into the world was one of the warmest feelings he'd ever had. Their courage and serenity touched him.

Knowing he needed more experience in plastic surgery, he arranged, with Franny's help, a six-month residency at the Memorial Hospital connected with the Sloan Kettering Cancer Institute in New York City. There, he began reconstructing deformities that came from removing facial or neck cancers in adults, as rewarding an experience as building new faces for children. He lived in a small room on the top floor of the New York hospital and became so lonely for Bobby and their two daughters that he vowed never again to be separated from them.

Each night, to help pass time, he wrote in his journal. Spilling out his thoughts onto paper, writing what he would not say in daylight, eased the day's frustrations or grievances. And, as he wrote, he would glance at the window to watch the twilight turn to night. The lights of the city spread a soft glow over the buildings.

Writing detailed notes on operations and conferences layered his days as if revisiting them. His notes offered up kernels of significance. He would then concentrate on the day ahead, writing down steps of scheduled surgeries. After going over and over each step, he soon had them "down cold," which became not just a rehearsal but a rootstock of confidence. Rehearsing, planning, and organizing were habits he'd formed in high school, and now they had become traits he depended on. At the same time, his mind was open to the need to adapt to the unforeseeable, to something that could come crashing in at any given moment. Every operation he now performed drew on those skills. And the surgeries were often tests of endurance lasting fourteen to sixteen hours.

Sitting alone at his desk at the top of the hospital, he often thought of his college and high school days, letting the memories ease some of his loneliness. Drifting in his thoughts was Thornton Wilder's play *Our Town*. He'd first seen it in high school. At other times, at different stages in his life, he's seen it in other theaters, in other cities. Always, the last act stayed with him—especially the scene in which the family's deceased daughter returns from her grave for one more day. Back in the town where she grew up, she finds her mother busy in the kitchen. She sees her brother and sisters getting ready for school. But none of them stop to take notice of her or of each other. Even as she begs them to see—even as she implores them to enjoy one another's company, to take note of the riches of their lives—no one listens. They pay attention only to their own interests, their own concerns. Sadly, she turns and returns to her grave.

Remembering that scene, Joe put down his pen. He walked downstairs into the rooms of the patients recovering in the wards. He checked them, looking for possible complications. He listened to their complaints. He listened to their worries and hopes. Realizing that he was seeing life in the raw, close to the very existence of being, as few are privileged to witness, he turned the moment over and over in his mind and held it still.

From then on, he would do the same each night: walk from room to room, check on those he took care of, connect with their most basic fears of illness, of death, of being in the grip of something they could not control.

———

When Joe had been discharged from the army in 1947, rumblings about transplantation were beginning to be heard in the margins of the medical community. Until then, the idea had pretty much been given up on. Rejection was viewed as too thick a barrier to break through. But with the knowledge of crush syndrome and the ability to keep those victims alive with blood transfusions, many surgeon-scientists began to reconsider transplanting an organ, specifically a kidney. And something else had happened to encourage the wild idea of borrowing organs. On a midnight in 1946 at the Brigham, a Hail Mary attempt to save a young woman's life became word-of-mouth proof that a human kidney could indeed be borrowed to preserve a life. No doubt Joe heard about it as soon as he returned to the Brigham from Valley Forge to finish his years of training. And the story fanned his curiosity first aroused by Charles's long-lasting skin grafts.

It began with a twenty-nine-year-old woman falling into a coma after an illegal abortion. The abortion had been performed without sterile precautions—which, unfortunately, was usual—and her uterus had been infected. She went into severe shock. Her blood pressure plunged; the flow of blood in her body became restricted, and her kidneys stopped working. Without producing any urine for ten days, her body was unable to excrete metabolic wastes as urine, and now she was moments from death.

As she was too sick to make it to the operating room, three doctors rushed her to a room at the end of the hall. There, by the light of two gooseneck lamps, they used a local anesthetic and attached the kidney of a patient who had just died to the young woman's arm.

Banking on what had been learned from crush syndrome, they hoped the cadaver kidney could carry her over until her injured kidneys might spontaneously begin to work. This was a year before Kolff visited the Brigham and left a blueprint of his dialysis machine, so that bridge was not available that night. And the three—a research fellow, the chief resident in urology, and the assistant resident in surgery—were willing to take the risk of borrowing a kidney for her. Grafting kidneys in animal models had been tried, but this operation would be the first attempt to borrow a human kidney to save a life. Throughout history, rejection had been the main barrier to transplantation, but another Herculean barrier lurked in the shadows. No one knew how to attach the organ to the veins and artery of the borrower's blood supply. Without a viable blood system to nourish the borrowed kidney, it would die. History was filled with half-baked ideas of transplanting limbs, blood, kidneys, skin—you name it—from one person to another. Always the results were heartbreaking, not just from rejection, but also from the inability to attach the organ to the recipient's blood supply. But the Brigham doctors were ready for that challenge: they intended to apply a fifty-year-old surgical technique discovered by Alexis Carrel in the early 1900s. They just didn't know if attaching a borrowed kidney to the borrower's blood supply would work.

Carrel's technique, known as *suture anastomosis*, was so universally appreciated that Carrel was awarded the Nobel Prize in 1912, a rare recognition for a surgeon. A Frenchman who had emigrated to the US, Carrel was inspired by the French art of making Valenciennes lace, using very fine needles and very thin threads of linen. He devised the technique at the University of Chicago and derived its name from the Greek *ana*, meaning *to*, and *stoma*, meaning *mouth*. The term literally means the joining of two round, hollow structures such as arteries.

Flamboyant with a desire for fame, Carrel had a long and dark history. For years he had transplanted limbs between dogs, kidneys between cats, and thyroids between various animals. He became famous for keeping a chicken heart beating in a culture medium, as if he had found the fountain of youth.

All of his transplanted organs failed because they were rejected by the host, which Carrel never understood. The transplants he could call successful had been done within the same animal, moving the kidneys to some other part of the animal's body, not from one to another. Because he had no understanding of the biological reasons for the rejection of foreign tissue, his transplanted organs rapidly stopped functioning. Yet his studies garnered attention, to the point of human patients begging him for help—one so desperate to live he asked Carrel to transplant a kidney from an executed criminal.

As he transplanted kidneys between dogs and cats, Carrel knew there was a biological force he did not understand and could not overcome. As each animal died when its transplant was rejected, Carrel insisted that the host was the reason, not the surgical factors. And he was partly right: suture anastomosis would last, and is still used today, especially in transplant surgery. But he also had significant blind spots, and in time his dark side took over as he became dedicated to proving the superiority of the white race and called for correcting "an error" in the US Constitution that promised equality for all people.

In 1928, Carrel collaborated with Charles Lindbergh in the development of a special kind of blood pump, which eventually informed the engineering of a method used in heart surgery. Carrel died in Europe awaiting trial for collaborating with the Nazis. His character flaws were prominent, but his method to successfully attach blood vessels lasted.

And on that night at the Brigham in 1946, his surgical technique would be soundly tested. If suture anastomosis could sustain blood flow to the borrowed human kidney, history would be made. Full of hope, the three doctors sewed the cadaver kidney into the arm of the dying woman, attaching it to the artery near her elbow and to the vein in front of it. With a kidney's blood supply coming from a single artery and vein, it made it a relatively straightforward organ to connect to the appropriate vessels—and a perfect organ to test the wild idea of transplantation.

Carrel's decades-old technique was working. No blood seeped through the sutured thread. When the three tried to bury the kidney beneath her skin, they were prevented by the position of the vessels, so a large part of the kidney was left exposed. They covered it with gauze and taped it to her arm. Only the tip of the ureter, which is normally the pathway into the bladder, was left exposed, and they positioned it in a laboratory flask where it could drain freely, and they could see it. That is, *if* the borrowed kidney worked. Then they waited. Hovering over her, they aimed the gooseneck lamps at the cadaver kidney to keep it warm. No doubt, they took note of the risk they had taken. If their innovative treatment failed, the woman's life would be lost for sure, and maybe that much more quickly. Furthermore, the criticism for doing this crazy thing could follow them, even affecting their careers. Yet the excitement of what they were doing could not be ignored. It was almost palpable in the small room.

Suddenly, the cadaver kidney dripped urine. Watching, mesmerized, the three were on the edge of celebration. The moment felt miraculous, even comic as they realized that such a basic human function could cause such joy! But joy it was, as the cadaver kidney kept working, drip by drip, and even gained steam, putting out more.

Watching over her, they stayed until it was nearly daylight. Only then did they leave to do their regular duties. By noon of the next day, the woman was alert. The borrowed kidney was still producing urine. Day two, the ureter swelled. Day three, the kidney decreased output, but the woman was so improved that the cadaver kidney was removed. Day four, the young woman was functioning normally. Soon, she walked out of the hospital into her reclaimed life. A first step had been taken; a new answer found.

This Hail Mary attempt—never published because it was just that, a risky, rogue procedure to save a life—became a legend passed from medical residents and professors to other residents and professors. When Franny heard of it, as chief of surgery, he was horrified that the procedure had been done outside of an operating room. Yet there was no disputing, no denying, that something important had been discovered. A borrowed kidney, attached by suture anastomosis, had functioned. This was a momentous leap in the new universe of transplantation, a move as significant as the one that would be taken more than twenty years later when a man stepped off a landing module onto the surface of the moon.

And even though Franny and Joe would never accept that comparison—they were too humble for that—what they would eventually achieve would be even greater than a moon landing. Theirs was a greater contribution to relieve suffering, a greater task to restore a life, a greater gift to mankind. That midnight treatment by those three risk-taking doctors showed that transplanting a human kidney was *not* crazy. It was, in fact, *doable*.

13

Not Exactly Cinderella's Mice

A MAGICAL MEETING was not on the calendar, but it was taking shape. In Britain, as Peter coaxed biology to give up its exquisite secrets, Joe and Franny were puzzling out transplantation's other barriers. When they were ready, they would ask Peter to come to the US to visit their labs and consult with them on their projects, enabling his life and work to intersect historically with that of Joe and Franny and others working at the Brigham.

Until then, Joe was finishing his training, knowing that plastic surgery would be a main interest. And as surgeon-scientists interested in transplantation, he and Franny were confronting three other significant unknowns: would a borrowed kidney remain healthy without its lymphatic supply? Could a transplanted organ function without nerves being attached to its new host? When a kidney was lifted from one body to another, would the transfer irreparably damage it?

No one knew.

In the lymphatic system, body fluids other than blood flow through organs with the lymphatic system's own network of vessels to return lymphocytes and proteins to the bloodstream. Since the kidney's lymphatic vessels are very small, so small that a borrowed organ could not be reconnected to the lymphatic vessels in a patient, could a transplanted kidney exist in its host unconnected to the lymphatic system? In other words, would sacrificing the lymphatic system affect a borrowed kidney?

Similarly, nerves leading to and from a borrowed organ, severed when it was removed, would be impossible to reattach in a host. Would the grafted kidney be okay?

A kidney is a living tissue. When physically moved from a donor to a host, would it be injured? How would you move it? Who should carry it? How much time would they have? And, always, the age-old problem of rejection remained.

In Britain, Peter was unveiling the workings of the immune system as it caused rejection. But it was a serendipitous meeting with a veterinarian that pushed his understanding of that biology into a new realm. That meeting, three years after the end of the war, was driven by his innate boldness.

Peter had never been one to indulge in himself even a hint of shyness. Dating back to his Oxford days, he liked to sit down beside someone he didn't know in order to match his restless mind against that of another, as if his thinking powers craved exercise. Such was the day he plunked himself down to have breakfast beside the famous writer C. S. Lewis and challenged him to a discussion of Jane Austen's novels. Right off, Lewis asked Peter, "What was the name of Mr. Woodhouse's butler?"

Irked, Peter had to admit he could not remember the butler's name but only how he boiled an egg. Already he was losing points in their mind match, but the final blow came when Lewis retorted, "Never discuss anything with an author except his royalties." Then he quipped, "From one as young as you are, to praise is as impertinent as to blame."

Undaunted, Peter chalked up the encounter as informative. When he later bumped into the poet T. S. Eliot on campus, he challenged the great man of letters right away to a discussion of novels. That didn't go well either when Eliot chose a novel to discuss that Peter had never read.

In 1948, Birmingham University's "boy professor" traveled to a meeting of international scientists in Stockholm. During a break, still undaunted about striking up a conversation with a stranger, Peter sat beside Hugh Donald, a Scottish veterinarian, introduced himself, and asked the man about his research. Donald was doing research on cattle twins only forty miles from Birmingham and immediately asked Peter if he knew a foolproof method of distinguishing between fraternal and identical cattle twins.

Apparently, solving that problem was important to the Agricultural Council in Edinburgh for producing cattle for food. Offhandedly, Peter answered, "My dear fellow, in principle the solution is extremely easy; exchange skin grafts between the twins and see how long they last. If they last indefinitely, you can be sure they are identical twins, but if they are thrown off, you can classify them with equal certainty as fraternal."

When Peter got home, he found a letter waiting for him from Donald, asking if he would come to the cattle farm to demonstrate the skin-graft technique to the research team. Feeling "morally obliged to comply," Peter said *yes*. After all, the farm was only forty miles away.

He asked his close friend and colleague Bill Billingham to drive up there with him. And together they performed a procedure similar to the grafting Peter had done in the past. He took a small piece of skin from one twin calf and grafted it onto the other. When all the grafts were done, and the usual period of waiting had passed to see which grafts were rejected to identify that twin as fraternal and not identical, Peter found the result astonishing. It was unlike

124

anything he had expected. All the cattle twins accepted each other's grafts as if the tissues were completely their own.

Of course, this result was not in line with what he knew about the natural history of skin grafts on all other animals. The only thing to do was to repeat the study immediately.

He and Bill were astonished when the results were the same. To help himself understand the outcome, Peter read about the work of the American geneticist Ray Owen in *The Production of Antibodies*, by Frank Burnet and Frank Fenner, which explored an elemental and critical phenomenon in the biology of the immune system: *tolerance*. Owen's work revealed that all cattle twins, fraternal or identical, have the same blood groups. Each twin has a mixture of blood corpuscles: those that are genetically its own and those that could have come only from its twin. The only way the twins could accept each other's tissues as their own would be if they were chimeras, that is, with a little of each in both. As for the Scottish cattle twins, the conclusion was that before birth they must have shared fused placentas.

Peter inferred that the cattle twins, as embryos in their mother's womb, were literally transfused with each other's blood during development. This sharing of fluids in the womb prepared them after birth to react to the other's tissues as if they were their own. *Antigens*, literally meaning "the things that generate antagonism," leaked from the yolk sack of each embryo into the sac of the other. Their intolerance of the other's tissues had been changed prior to birth.

Peter was onto a new way of thinking: *tolerance could be acquired.* The pre-birth stage of development held answers. Already, studies at Stanford University in 1929 had proven that when grafting different colored feathers onto newly hatched Rhode Island Red and Plymouth Rock chickens, the cells that were transplanted were accepted, while no transplants survived on older birds with a more mature immune system.

As Peter was looking into other studies of the pre-birth phenomenon, he found that another creative scientist, Milan Hašek, had discovered the same outcome. Hašek, who lived in Czechoslovakia, showed that the circulations of chick embryos united *in utero* produced mature chickens able to accept each other's skin grafts without rejection. His research was cutting edge. He and Peter soon became enthusiastic colleagues sharing their findings. They were both battering the rejection barrier toward the magical moment when human biology would be understood well enough to exchange not just skin, but an organ.

It was already known that certain places in the body, such as the anterior chamber of the eye, were free of the immune process. A transplant there would not be attacked. These were considered "privileged sites." So now Peter surmised that in the case of other tissues, there must be "a privileged time" for transplantation, such as pre-birth.

He then undertook the next step in unlocking the secrets of the immune system.

And he did so with passion.

Turning science on its head, he was about to prove the possibility of not just going *around* the natural barrier that prohibits transplanting foreign tissues, but actually *breaking* it. This was revolutionary, indeed. For years, a significant number of scientists maintained that breaking down the immunological barrier was in principle impossible, that the substances that stimulate normal rejection are part of a body's genetic makeup. In this view, a person's immune system barrier was as unchangeable as a blood group.

Peter considered his discovery of tolerance to be not only practical but moral. If he could further his proof that immunity could be manipulated, he would give heart to those surgeon-scientists who dreamed of saving a life by transplanting an organ. He would push the infant field of transplantation studies into an orbit yet unimagined.

Now his life and family were taken over with families of mice. As Peter undertook studies to turn them into manufactured chimeras, to make them able to wear different colors of fur patches with no rejection, he aimed to display the same memory biology as identical twins. His mice were not exactly Cinderella's mice, but they *were* about to become world famous.

———————

RUNNING EXPERIMENTS ON animals is contentious. Peter had been using animal models for most of his scientific career and was involved in maintaining regulations for doing so with compassionate oversight. The practice—known as vivisection (cutting on live animals)—dates back to antiquity and, in time, became a moral dilemma when animals were depicted in paintings as having human-like emotions. For those of us who find animal companionship to be one of the sweetest delights as we share the earth with a variety of species, the use of animal models in research is particularly agonizing.

Perhaps the best illustration of the conflict is the realization that without some seventeen thousand monkeys, imported from India and housed in a special farm in South Carolina, Jonas Salk would not have been able to find the three different strains of the poliovirus and create the 1954 vaccine that could build immunity to those strains, one of which attacked thirty to fifty thousand children a year, with paralyzing effects.

From the moment that humans discovered their own curiosity, they began cutting into the bodies of living animals for scientific research. But it was not until universities began endorsing the method of turning to animals as models for scientific investigation, as well as for teaching, that such use of animals became traditional.

A turning point was the published findings of the French physiologist François Magendie on the function of the spinal cord. He used cruel practices on research animals that provoked a public outcry. Afterward, anesthetizing animals for procedures in the research lab became a common practice. And a significant shift came in the late 1800s, when medical schools began using animal models in teaching their students anatomy and physical diagnosis. Universities then established their own animal laboratories and hired physiologists to run them.

With more animals being used in science and medicine, the need for standardized restrictions became obvious. *The Handbook for the Physiological Laboratory* was published in 1873, setting forth the rules to be followed.

In the eighteenth and nineteenth centuries, many began to think of animals not just as "beasts of burden" but as beings that should be valued and protected. Artists and writers began raising the public's awareness. William Hogarth's painting *Four Stages of Cruelty* graphically depicted animal suffering. Even Mary Shelley, in her masterpiece *Frankenstein*, wrote that the monster's creator had "tortured the living animal to animate the lifeless clay." The poet Alexander Pope and essayist Joseph Addison also weighed in on the issue. And during Queen Victoria's reign other humanist issues were embraced, and the antivivisectionist movement spread worldwide.

On New York City streets, citizens watched with concern as horses fell from fatigue and malnutrition. The outcry was loud enough that the American Society for the Prevention of Cruelty to Animals was formed, which in turn led to a hard look at the ways in which children were treated and to laws against child abuse.

The dilemma of using animals in research was especially clarified by the outcry of dog lovers against Louis Pasteur's work on a rabies vaccine. While dog lovers protested, Pasteur not only discovered the means to save an endless number of dogs' lives from hideous suffering, his studies also led to protecting their owners from a disease so dangerous it led to insanity and death. And today, rabies vaccines are required by law. Diseases that affect both humans and animals illuminate the interconnectedness of creatures who share the earth.

The National Institutes of Health in the United States, with other federal agencies, began setting current regulations. In Britain, Peter oversaw the restrictions for using animal models in research, soon requiring that laboratories have licenses. In Joe's lab at the Brigham, and in the labs of other scientists studying the implantation of kidney bridges into patients dying of renal failure, the hero subjects for the surgical rehearsals were creatures whose vessel and vein dimensions most resembled those of a human. Eventual fame would come to canine transplant pioneers in the Brigham lab named Sam, Honest John, New Hampshire, and Mona.

Peter's mice subjects, however, offered a different story. Living for a while in the Medawar household, in many ways they took over the family's life. Each of Peter and Jean's four children, whom Peter biblically called "olives around his table," took a family of elegant brown and white mice to live in their rooms. They ran up and down each child while Jean and Peter watched, laughing. In the mornings the whole Medawar family sat in rapt silence and delight watching their mice families perform their daily chores of spitting, combing, and polishing themselves. They even fluffed up the wood shavings of their beds.

Before taking up their careers in Peter's lab, these household mice took on the names that Jean, Peter, and their children gave them. Going down the alphabet, their names were Anonymous, Bigamous and Blasphemous, Dormouse, Enormous, Famous, Infamous, Lachrymose, Magnanimous (Peter's favorite), until they got to Posthumous, which Jean said should stop the line.

Each played a part in Peter's research as he set about exploring what he had learned from the cattle twins. His goal was to swap fur, to have a black mouse wear a white patch, and a white mouse have a black patch—each without rejecting the skin tissue infused with color. The process would take time; what Peter called the body's exquisite power would not be a simple nut to crack. He was peeling back the layers of its mysteries a little at a time.

Unveiling the immune system's secrets was his life's work. If you asked him, he surely would have replied—as any who signed on to serve during World War II to keep Nazism from invading democracies around the world—that, of course, he was willing to give his life for science to offer up its truths.

14

"Give the Kid a Chance"

BY THE END OF JUNE 1950, Joe had finished his sixth-month rotation in plastic surgery that Franny had arranged for him at Memorial Hospital in New York. And he knew now—with no doubts—that he was going to pursue a career as a plastic surgeon. To become board certified, he needed another year of training, this time at New York Hospital across from Memorial.

Since the thought of being separated from his young family any longer was unbearable, he found an apartment ten minutes from the hospital. And Bobby, the girls, and the new baby on the way joined him there. By now he knew that family came first. Without Bobby and their children, he was adrift, unable to be at his best.

As 1951 arrived, Joe was winding up his last year in training and by the following July was back in Boston, ready to start private practice. Dr. Bradford Cannon took him on as a clinical associate and gave him space in his office on Dartmouth Street.

That first year, Joe had a total of three patients. He was also in debt for an examining table that he compared to a custom-made Ferrari. He kept busy as a plastic surgical consultant, accompanying Dr. Cannon on his hospital rounds to four hospitals. Each week, there were also tumor clinics at two veterans' hospitals to attend. With his experience at Valley Forge and the New York hospitals, he felt ahead of the other surgeons. But he bit his tongue.

Sitting on his impatience, he waited. One day at a tumor conference, the surgeons at the conference table asked him how he would treat a man who had just come in with an extensive tongue cancer invading his jawbone. Joe had done just such a case while at New York Hospital. He laid out the procedures he had used to excise the cancer and perform immediate reconstruction. Usually reconstruction was performed in a later, separate operation, which, to Joe, made no sense. Do it all at once he thought; build back a face during the same surgery, as he had learned to do at Valley Forge.

When he finished laying out his plan for the patient, Dr. Cannon jumped in, saying, "Give the kid a chance." Joe suspected Dr. Cannon must have briefed the chief of surgery on his frustration, for now the chief quickly echoed, "How about we give the young fellow a chance to show what he can do?"

Joe performed the surgery. He took out the tumor and used a bone graft to replace the excised part of the jawbone. A week later, when he returned to Veterans Hospital, the staff greeted him as a hero. No one expected the patient to recover from such extensive surgery without serious complications.

Joe's specialized practice was now launched.

No plastic surgery service existed at the Brigham; a weekly visit from the plastic surgeon at Children's Hospital was serving the Brigham's needs. When Franny invited Joe to treat patients there, he jumped at the chance. In joining the staff, he would not only be doing plastic surgery as well as general surgery, he would also be allowed to explore his seemingly off-the-wall idea of kidney transplantation. Already in place at the Brigham was a program for the treatment of kidney disease, with hospital administrators, physicians, surgeons, pathologists, radiologists, nurses, and social workers ready to take on the unprecedented effort of treating end-stage renal disease with a groundbreaking approach.

There were warnings, though. Many called organ transplantation science fiction, a field for fools. Joe was told that he could harm his career. If organ transplantation was viewed as a risky field only for the foolhardy, Joe was more than happy to sign on as a member. Despite the seemingly miraculous invention of the dialysis machine, its limits were becoming heartbreakingly clear. Dialysis could keep a patient alive for only so long, and as those with chronic, ongoing kidney failure were kept alive for weeks, months, or even a year, without the hope of replacing their diseased kidneys there was no future to look forward to.

In March 1951, that exact situation led to the first desperate and remarkable attempt to transplant a kidney. A thirty-seven-year-old man came to the Springfield Hospital with his kidneys failing. His surgeon, James Scola, asked the Brigham to accept him for dialysis. As a child, the man had developed glomerulonephritis after a severe streptococcal sore throat. The dangerous bacterium that often causes strep throat can be cured with penicillin, but when the man contracted strep as a child, penicillin was not available to the general public. Now that early bout of strep had left damage to his kidneys, and that damage threatened his life.

At the Brigham, he received dialysis, which improved his condition. But his well-being was only temporary. Every day he moved closer to death. He went back to the Springfield Hospital with no future, no hope, and no options. When Dr. Scola told him that a nearby dying patient had offered his kidney on the chance it could be transplanted, the man jumped at the idea.

In groundbreaking surgery, Dr. Scola placed the donor kidney in his desperate patient, attaching its blood supply by the intricate suture anastomosis devised by Alexis Carrel decades before. The borrowed kidney was without a blood supply for seventy minutes.

The Brigham transplant team closely followed this historic first try. After surgery, the patient was sent back to the Brigham where the transplant team could care for him with the dialysis machine standing by. For a few days, he did well. But the output from the transplanted kidney was meager, certainly not enough to maintain a normal life. Dialysis could not relieve his progressing renal failure, and five weeks after the risk-taking surgery, he died.

During an autopsy, the borrowed kidney was found to be surrounded by infection, showing all the changes associated with rejection.

Three weeks later, refusing to give up, the Brigham transplant team decided to try a different tactic. Kidney transplantation now appeared the only option to relieve not only suffering, but an end to the added suffering of having no hope to live without it. In April 1951, the Brigham surgical team designed a new trial. They placed kidneys in the upper thighs of patients being kept alive only by dialysis.

Placing a kidney in the thigh required only local anesthesia. Furthermore, the transplanted kidney could easily be monitored and, if found to be harming the patient, easily removed. These kidneys came from within the hospital as by-products of surgery for hydrocephalus, also known also "water on the brain." In children the condition is usually caused by a congenital abnormality, leading to an accumulation of too much fluid in the ventricles of the brain. A former classmate of Franny, Don Matson, had advanced a procedure to relieve the pressure by placing a small plastic tube, a shunt, to drain the fluid from the child's brain into the ureter, out through the bladder. In that way, the excess fluid was flushed from the child's body along with urine. In placing the shunt, the surgery required that one kidney had to be sacrificed.

Don's support was critical. Franny had asked him to see if the children's parents would donate the sacrificed kidneys to the transplant trials. After all, he and Don were bonded from their mischief-making days when Don put on a grass skirt to spoof the Harvard Medical School faculty in a skit. That Franny asked Don to supply kidneys for their new trial made a lot of sense. In the 1940s, Don had supplied spare kidneys for vaccine research, sending them across the street to Boston Children's Hospital, where a team of residents led by Dr. John Enders was trying to grow viruses in tissue culture with the goal of producing vaccines to prevent them. One day Enders and his residents Weller and Robbins put various viruses, along with the poliovirus, in one of Don's donated human kidney tissues and, astonished, watched it begin to grow. There was the answer that Jonas Salk had been searching for: kidney tissue could become the means to produce the virus to harvest for a vaccine. The discovery led to Enders and his residents being awarded the Nobel Prize in 1954.

During the war, Don had served close to the front lines, collecting information for new surgical treatments for brain injuries, which he then summarized for the surgeon general. Eventually he would become famous for publishing the first comprehensive text on the neurosurgery of infancy and childhood. His residents looked upon him with awe and trepidation, but with really no need. He had such a mild temperament that he would often nudge aside a resident in the midst of surgery, saying gently, "Let me take a look for a minute." When Joe and Franny asked him to participate in the thigh-kidney trials, he was happy to oblige and passed along sacrificed kidneys to give hope to those dying of renal failure.

For a while, those kidneys worked well. They held good color. They made urine. But within days, things changed. The kidneys lost color. They shriveled and stopped putting out urine. The patient showed signs of battling rejection and soon died.

Dejected, the surgeon-scientists assessed what the trials had made clear. Rejection was more complicated than anyone had guessed. Joe and Franny took comfort in reminding themselves that "a start must be made if anything at all is to be achieved."

Now they were back to square one.

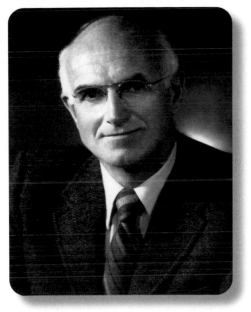

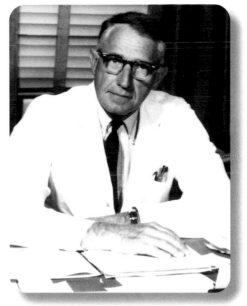

Dr. Joseph Edward Murray

Dr. Francis Daniels Moore

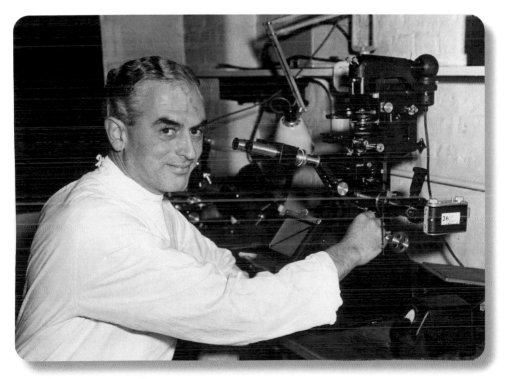

Sir Peter Brian Medawar

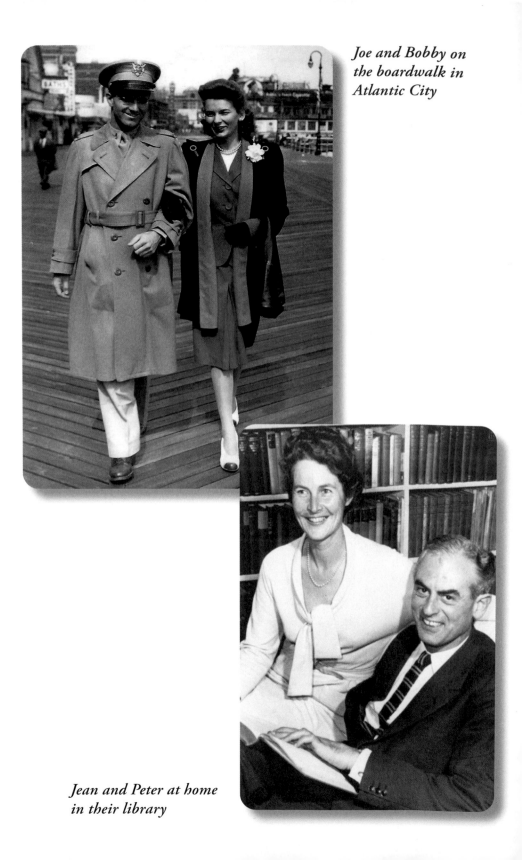

Joe and Bobby on the boardwalk in Atlantic City

Jean and Peter at home in their library

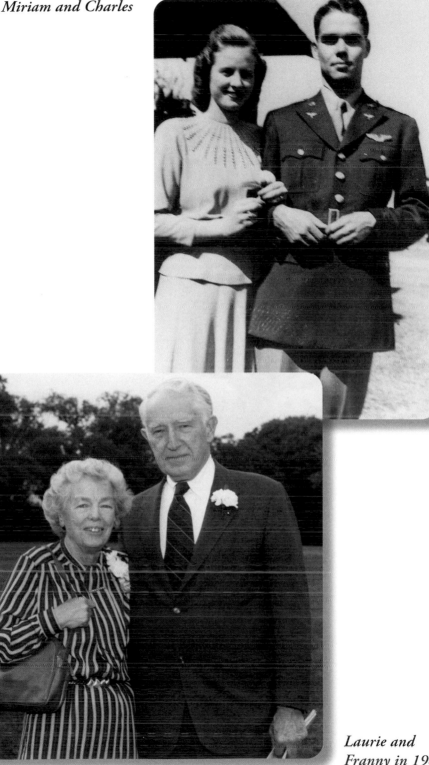

Miriam and Charles

*Laurie and
Franny in 1982*

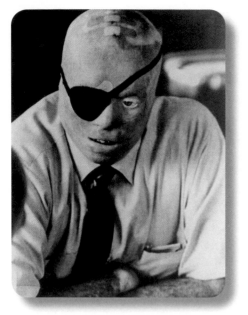

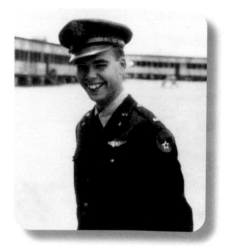

Charles Woods in uniform, not long before taking on the challenge of "Flying the Hump"

Charles Woods, during his campaign for governor of Alabama in 1970

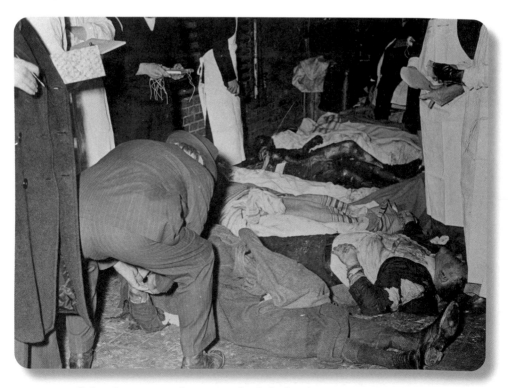

Victims of the Cocoanut Grove Nightclub fire lying in a Boston morgue. Note the sailor, left, holding identification tags to be placed on the bodies.

Richard (left) and Ronald Herrick, leaving Peter Bent Brigham Hospital in January 1955, fully recovered

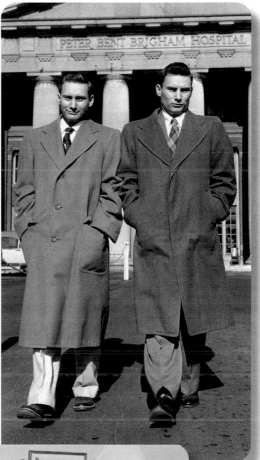

Ronald Herrick showing a nurse a picture of his twin, Richard, in the coast guard

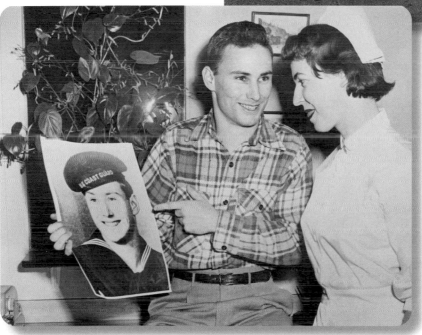

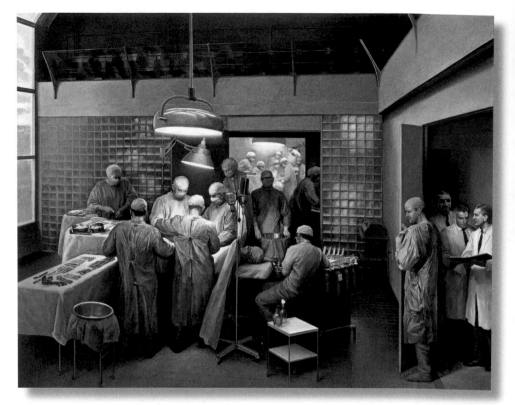

Joel Babb's painting of the first successful organ transplant.
This beautiful piece now hangs in the Harvard Medical Library
in the Francis A. Countway Library of Medicine in Boston.

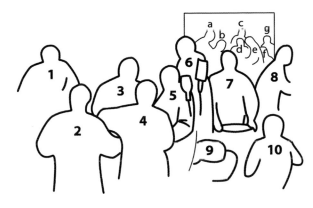

1. **Mrs. Maxine Rhodes** – Scrub Nurse

2. **Daniel Edgar Pugh** – Surgical Intern

3. **Joseph Edward Murray** – Transplant Surgeon

4. **John Loring Rowbotham** – Chief Resident Surgeon

5. **Edward Barton Gray** – Surgical Resident

6. **Mrs. Elizabeth Comiskey** – Circulating Nurse

7. **Francis Daniels Moore** – Chief of Surgery

8. **Extra Scrub Nurse** – Fictional

9. **Richard Herrick** – Recipient Patient

10. **Leroy David Vandam** – Anesthesiologist

11. **John Hartwell Harrison** – Urological Surgeon

12. **Gustave John Dammin** – Chief Pathologist

13. **John Putnam Merrill** – Nephrologist

14. **George Widmer Thorn** – Chief of Medicine

a. **Miss Alice Maxwell** – Scrub Nurse

b. **John Hartwell Harrison** – Urological Surgeon, shown again

c. **Miss Marian Wheet** – Circulating Nurse

d. **Robert Austin Milch** – Junior Surgical Resident

e. **Murray Benjamin Pincus** – Chief Resident, Urology

f. **Charles Peter Crowe** – Surgical Intern, Anesthesia Rotation

g. **Thomas Kelvin Burnap** – Anesthesiologist

The full names, clinical roles, and signatures of all participants involved in the two surgical procedures associated with the world's first successful organ transplant

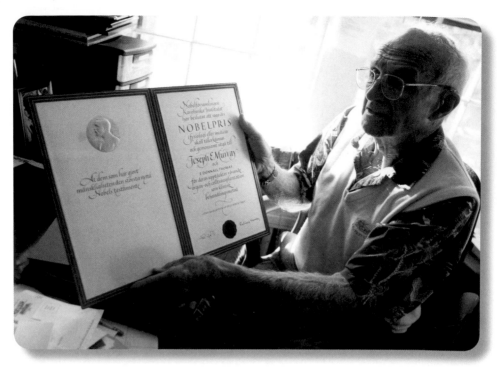

Joe Murray showing his Nobel Prize citation

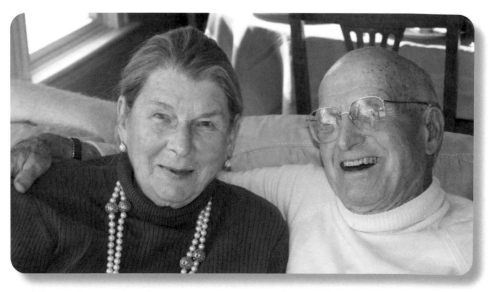

Bobby and Joe, Thanksgiving Day 2012. That night Joe would suffer the stroke that ended his life.

15

"My Mind, You Know, Never Lets Me Rest"

IN 1951, four years after being made dean and professor at the University of Birmingham, Peter was invited to submit his name for the Jodrell Chair of Zoology at the University of London. It was the longest established chair of zoology in England, carrying great prestige.

He applied and was elected. His partner, Bill Billingham, who had pioneered the work on the cattle twins with him, was willing to move to London to continue the research they were doing. So a new chapter in all their lives was about to begin.

The move promised to be complicated; the Medawars now had a large family, not just of pets and children but also of parents and in-laws who visited often. Jean was worried about finding a suitable house with space for everyone. One morning, while she was folding a sheet of *The Times* to line a drawer, she saw an ad: *Queen Anne–period house with garden in Hampstead.* Immediately she got on the train to London, saw the house—four floors near the underground rail line to the University of London and to the 880 acres of Hampstead Heath. Instantly, she made an offer. Then she went home and sold their car to afford it. For the next year, she and Peter were carless, but the house was worth it. And they were now settled in London.

Peter's talent for administration was unexpected, though he vowed never to let it get in the way of his science. By gathering stimulating colleagues around him, he created what he called a "matey" feeling, an atmosphere he felt was essential to fruitful research. No time was wasted in rivalry or intrigue. Authors' names on published material were arranged alphabetically, not by precedence. Colleagues played squash together. They spent time in pubs debating ideas.

Peter took up smoking. He also bore down on his important research, which he jokingly called the "period of the supermice." He reproduced what he had observed in the cattle twins by performing a simple operation that did not interfere with gestation. Through the body wall of a brown mouse female, he delicately injected her embryos with living cells from one of the white mice. Peter and his colleagues eventually found the right dose of these "foreign non-self" cells, as well as their right state of development, that allowed the mouse embryo to accept them.

As adults, those mice were then given skin grafts from mice of the opposite color. After trial and error, Peter finally had a population of living mice running around in solid-colored fur interrupted with an opposite-colored patch. The normal time span of transplanted tissue, ten to twelve days, came and went. No rejection. He had produced the tolerance he had witnessed in the twin cattle. Exposing unborn mice to the foreign cells of another so early in life "fooled" them into accepting these transplanted cells as "self."

The mice families lived in big, round glass containers with sawdust bottoms and a perforated lid at Peter's lab at the university. He liked to watch them, finding them much more intelligent than most humans think. He saw how they learned to stand on their hind legs to dislodge the lid and compromise the security Peter had counted on.

By then, a pack of street mice had found a hole in the laboratory floorboards and moved in, living as squatters, until one of the priceless laboratory mice sprang from his container and disappeared down the street-mice hole. Hearing squeaks, scuffles, and flopping, Peter knew a terrific battle was underway. All he could do was hope for the best and root for his mouse with its multicolored coat.

After a few minutes, his valuable research mouse crawled up through the hole. It stood panting with a torn ear before collapsing. Peter said it breathed its last as a hero to science.

These studies demonstrated that the immune system could indeed be manipulated prior to birth, but Peter knew he had to duplicate the study in another animal model. He decided to repeat the work of Milan Hašck, the gifted Czechoslovakian biologist. Hašek had accomplished a union between two chicken embryos and found that the chicken twins hatched from this union were tolerant of each other's red blood cells. Soon, Peter had his own second-generation chimeric chickens—artificially produced twin chicks—strutting around his lab, carrying healthy living tissues from chicks that were genetically different. And no chicken had ill effects or obvious signs of being altered before birth.

By duplicating Hašek's findings, Peter added to his body of work. For years, he had carefully and clearly displayed the workings of the immune system. He was nearly ready to publish his groundbreaking research, which he would call the beauty and wonder of science.

His findings had yielded two brilliant discoveries. First, the second set phenomenon: the body's ability to recognize a second invasion of a protein with greater vigor than the first introduction of a foreign protein—a discovery that applied to all vertebrates such as birds, mammals, and primates. The other was his brilliant study in manipulating embryos prior to birth, proving that the immunological barrier could indeed be broken. He had shown there was a *privileged time* for the transplantation of a foreign tissue. The commingling of fluids between two unborn organisms led to their being able to accept, as adults, each other's foreign tissues with no rejection. Pre-birth manipulation equipped an organism to recognize transplanted tissue as "self."

The challenge now for Joe and Franny would be to apply this basic science to human biology.

IN THE UNITED STATES, the Rockefeller Institute, as the foremost center for biomedical research in the world, sought brilliant scientists to spend time in America to exchange ideas. Peter's eminence in immunology was now such that the institute invited him to give a series of lectures at Harvard. He came to the United States for the first time in September 1949. As soon as he walked off the ocean liner SS *Mauretania*, he stood on a New York City street and looked up. The height of the buildings astonished him. Coming from Britain, still in the midst of postwar austerity, he was even more impressed by the display of American wealth.

Peter also realized that it was "not a good moment in American history." The country was in the throes of the anti-intellectual fervor spawned by the speeches of Senator Joseph McCarthy. By the time of Peter's visit, all areas of American life were suspected of being infiltrated by communists. When Peter applied for a visa at the American consulate in London and was asked if he had any intentions of overthrowing the constitution of the United States, he answered with an Oxford man's cheekiness: he had no such purpose, but "if I were to do it by mistake I should be inexpressively contrite."

Fortunately, he was admitted anyway.

Mesmerized by automats and their remarkable ability to spew out an inexpensive meal, Peter ate in them all the time, saving enough money to send for Jean, who traveled over on the *Queen Mary*, fell out of her bed during a storm, and considered it all great fun.

Peter met her at the dock and rushed her to Rockefeller Center, which disappeared into the clouds. She bent her head back to spy the tip, sending her sealskin hat to the sidewalk. As soon as it was back on, Peter rushed her to witness the miracle of an automat.

Even though Cold War tactics were beginning to affect the international scientific community, Peter continued working without intellectual constraint. Fortunately, too, the clamp on academic freedom for those behind the Iron Curtain had not yet stopped the burgeoning field of immunology. Scientists were crying out for new data, new technologies, and a fresh point of view.

Peter was ready to provide that point of view. Building on prior research, he was refashioning past knowledge into a new world of science, reinvigorated by what had been learned from treating war wounds. Funding from the United States and from private foundations was flowing to British scientists. He often said that being a scientist felt like being "born anew every morning." And once he confided to a colleague, "My mind, you know, never lets me rest." To which his colleague quickly added, "or anyone else."

At the age of only thirty-four, he was visiting America as a foremost thinker in an increasingly clear universe of science that had always been a foggy, confusing puzzle. In the Harvard lecture hall that September, he paced up and down the stage, using almost no notes. He described his scientific studies as if recounting a game's sudden-death playoff. His audience of scientists was virtually hypnotized by his skill at turning dry academic information into the stuff of riveting mystery.

His life's first great challenge, he liked to say, was overcoming the worldview of his nanny, Winnie, who each Sunday read to him any newspaper articles that recounted the week's rapes, murders, batteries, arsons, and marital infidelities in high places. By the time he was twelve, he needed an antidote.

Love, the great remedy for what he called *pubescent dyspepsia*, saved him. And it came in the form of a stack of records from the golden age of opera in his parents' living room. He would put one of their records on their windup gramophone with its seven-foot horn, turn up the volume, and blast *Madame Butterfly* to the ceiling. Listening, his heart grew warm, and his enthusiasm for life, which nanny Winnie had nearly decapitated, returned. From then on, each week he saved his money to buy another record to rush home and play. His love for the dramatic was born.

As opera drew out emotions he didn't even know he had, he began memorizing songs from his favorites. His standards were from *Il Trovatore* and *Madame Butterfly*, which he sang, even though he could not sing. Later, as a student at his English public school, he found a classmate, John Vincent Godefroy, who shared his love. Though he owned the barrel chest of a baritone, Godefroy would let loose in a penetrating falsetto. He and Peter memorized parts of *Aida* and sang them to the horror of their classmates. Later, when one of these listeners was a student at Cambridge, he said that hearing the Medawar-Godefroy duo was one of the most terrible experiences he had ever lived through. Digesting the criticism, Peter said, "Well, you can't please everybody," and transferred his opera-singing to the shower.

While courting Jean, he introduced her to his favorite records, and after their marriage, while they listened to the sounds coming from the long golden horn of the gramophone or the stage of a concert hall, he would grip her fingers so tightly that her wedding ring left imprints. Jean silently watched as tears ran down his face. On occasion, he even sobbed.

On stage, describing his work, his flair for the dramatic took flight. His passion and dedication to the beauty of science and its quest for truth were riveting. He delivered ideas for new medical treatments with a unique ability to melt the barriers between basic scientists and clinicians. He described his studies clearly, almost like scientific recipes. Hearing him, scientists couldn't wait to get home and get started on their own ideas.

He made it clear in those American lectures that, with regard to the immune system, one simple concept needed to be understood, accepted, and employed, especially in the dream factory of transplantation that was spreading around the medical world. He emphasized the imperative understanding that the immune system had a *memory*—that our bodies rack up memories at a cellular level. Furthermore, it was a biological memory set up to rarely, if ever, fail. He liked to demonstrate the problem that the immune system presented to transplantation by saying, simply, that the body could not discern its friends from its enemies.

He proposed the question that if rejection was an allergic or immunological process, then couldn't it also be manipulated? And, if so, shouldn't organ tissue, such as a kidney, be able to be transplanted to save unimagined numbers of lives? All that was needed were those central missing answers: how does one manipulate the immune system? How does one prevent damage to an organ as it is taken from one to be given to another? How does one surgically place it and attach the vessels?

The puzzle pieces were ready to fall into place.

16

"By the Way, This Patient Has an Identical Twin"

As THE 1950s BEGAN, answers to the workings of the body's immune system were imminent. So was the fascinating technology of television and how the transmission of beams could connect Americans and people across the globe. In 1948, the organizers of the Republican National Convention hired engineers to put an antenna in a B-29 and send it twenty-five thousand feet above Pittsburgh, from where it transmitted the political event to viewers in nine American cities.

In another three years, a grid of ground cable enabled President Truman's 1951 speech at the Treaty of Peace with Japan to become the first coast-to-coast television broadcast. Carried by ninety-four stations to forty million viewers, the broadcast opened a new window in American culture. Soon, networks signed up local channels, and the shift from radio to television was on its way.

Charles Woods was buying up radio and television stations. Peter Medawar was publishing his groundbreaking research. Joe Murray was spending hours in the operating room and in his lab. Transplanting kidneys in dogs allowed him to perfect the surgical techniques he would need for a human transplant, while also answering crucial questions of how and where to place a borrowed organ. Franny Moore was digesting the basic science findings, especially Peter's, toward the dream of transplanting a kidney, realizing that a successful surgery would make medical history at the Brigham. He was also carrying out his own research on wellness care of the surgical patient, pioneering a technique of using radioactive isotopes (a blend of chemical elements) to locate abscesses and tumors. All the while, he was writing chapters in his textbook *Metabolic Care of the Surgical Patient*, which would be published at the end of the decade.

Franny took note of a curious case in England in 1950, when three five-year-old boys were suspected of having been incorrectly identified in the newborn nursery. Two were thought to be identical twins. To determine their true identities, small patches of skin from each were traded among the three with the assumption that the skin between the identical twins would be accepted perfectly, while the third unrelated child would reject it. This was the first time that skin grafts had been used as a form of establishing identity. And the outcome allowed the boys to be restored to their rightful parents. This case would prove to be vital to the moment when, in only four years, Joe would walk into the operating room to make history by successfully transplanting a kidney. Knowing with little doubt that the donor and recipient were perfect biological matches could mean the difference between failure and a page in history.

Science was the bedrock that the Brigham transplant team was relying on. And that science was adding up.

In 1951, Peter and Billingham lost no time publishing their first findings, authored with colleagues Anderson and Lampkin, in a newly established journal of genetics, *Heredity*. The article was titled "The use of skin grafting to distinguish between monozygotic and dizygotic twins," soon to become known as the phenomenon *tolerance*.

Two years later, with Billingham and Leslie Brent, Peter published an astonishingly short three-and-a-half-page article titled

"Actively acquired tolerance of foreign cells" in the October 3, 1953, issue of *Nature*. It was a blinding discovery. It also reached a worldwide audience, notably published in the same journal, same volume, as Watson and Crick's groundbreaking discovery that the genetic code for the development of an individual comes from a chemical, deoxyribonucleic acid (DNA), the building blocks of life. That two contributions to the well-being of mankind would be published at the same time in the same journal was a stunning awakening to a new age of vigorous scientific exploration. It was also a celebration of the creative minds at work changing the world.

————————

TRANSPLANT STUDIES IN ENGLAND, Scotland, Denmark, and Australia were vigorous. The world of medicine knew by now that transplantation was a universe open for exploration. It wasn't that a race had begun for performance of the first successful surgery, but certainly there was an awareness that the first to do it would make a mark on history. Franny, always keeping up with what was happening, noted that "about 1950, some French workers had removed kidneys from recently guillotined criminals and placed them in patients chronically ill with uremia." Of course, the outcome was dreadful, but the sensation of it caught attention, alerting the world that the giving and taking of organs could become reality in a future speeding toward them.

Then the Brigham made its own mark with a series of near misses. On October 17, 1952, a twenty-six-year-old doctor was admitted to the Brigham with chronic glomerulonephritis. He had high blood pressure, swelling of his ankles, headaches, and difficulty with his vision. He was in advanced kidney failure. On February 11, 1953, a new kidney was placed in his right thigh.

The donated kidney came from a young woman who had just died during a heart operation. When her blood type was found to be compatible with that of the sick doctor, her family was comforted by knowing they could donate her organ. After the transplant, the borrowed kidney made no urine; a large blood clot formed around it. The polyethylene bag used to protect it from the environment developed a tear. For a while, things looked dark, very dark. Then, on the nineteenth day, the kidney produced increasing amounts of urine. Six days later, it was making urine every day.

The doctor-patient handled infection, bleeding, and total kidney failure. But his wounds healed, and the transplanted kidney in his thigh still worked. He got out of bed and began to walk around. His blood counts showed that his body was *not* fighting the "foreign" kidney. After eighty-one days, he was released to go home.

This was the first time a human lived solely on the function of a kidney taken from another.

Yet, despite careful monitoring and supreme care, the young doctor suddenly died. The autopsy revealed that he expired as much from heart as from kidney failure. Interestingly, there was little evidence of rejection. Instead, the kidney graft's arteries had hardened. The patient had lived 175 days with good kidney function, while none of the others in the new trial of kidney grafts placed in the thigh experienced that length of success.

The team's surgeon-scientists, including Joe, now speculated that some close genetic relationship must have existed between the woman who died on the operating table and the physician who received her kidney. All theories pointed to there being some unexpected compatibility. Joe noted that transplanted tissue was "rejected with a vigor proportional to the degree of the genetic disparity" between donor and recipient.

Yes, compatibility—that was the key.

Peter's research had already shown that what happened pre-birth was the predictor for exchanging tissue without rejection. Franny noted that the good result of the doctor's case "must remain a mystery," and that "some of nature's creatures are more closely related to each other than might appear on the surface—a sort of random tissue-resemblance."

Clearly, kinship was the enigma to be explored and understood, the foremost factor in a successful kidney transplant.

When the surgeon-scientist directing these transplant trials, Dr. David Hume, left the Brigham for another appointment, Joe assumed responsibility for exploring the best way to do a kidney graft. His lab would soon become a zone of vigorous innovation.

He spent each Tuesday and Thursday in his laboratory, practicing transplant surgical techniques on animal models. He often stayed until midnight so he would not get behind in his regular surgical schedule. Each morning at five he would rise and dress in the house that he and Bobby had bought in a suburb of Boston. As their family grew from one child to two, from two to three, aiming for an eventual six, the size of their house grew too.

Each morning, Joe ate his burned toast while hanging over the sink, brushing off the black top layer, which he called soot. Then he got into his car—always a convertible, always with the top down in any weather, except torrential rain. Driving in a snowstorm, however, was appropriate for someone born on April Fool's Day. By 5:45, he was on Route 9 cruising toward Huntington Avenue and Brigham Circle, which led to the hospital.

All the way, he waved to the other commuters driving the same route, also aiming to be at their workplaces by a little after six o'clock. They became a community in motion, fellow commuters on a shared timeline.

By now, Bobby was calling Joe "Pollyanna." Their family life was everything. No television in the house. Kids fighting and wrestling on the living room rug, often with Joe among them. When the noise and hullabaloo reached the level of a sonic boom, Joe told everyone to go somewhere alone and read a book. And always music and singing filled the house. The kids took piano lessons, practicing early in the mornings before school. Each was also assigned chores that had to be completed with no complaining.

On those days when he was in his lab, Joe worked with basic scientists. And, of course, there were the problems that only he, as a surgeon, could address: where in the body should a transplanted kidney be placed? Should the diseased kidneys be removed? How should one handle the tissue in transport from the donor to the recipient? In some organs, cells are formed into sheets working from the same blood supply, whereas in the kidney, cells are functionally precise with many different kinds of cells. Transplanting those working cells would mean they could not be damaged during the movement of the organ from one body to another. But infection was the enemy in any surgery, and transplant surgery would be no exception. Always, there was the off chance that nature could throw in a complication, like an unexpected heart condition, a virus, or something as yet unimagined.

By now Joe and Franny, thanks to Peter's research, knew that for the first attempt to successfully transplant cellular tissues, a kidney, in a human, three conditions had to be in place. (1) They had to have a *privileged situation* to prevent the antibodies from getting at the grafted kidney, as Peter's cattle studies had proven. (2) They would have to change the tissue of the kidney itself so that it was no longer antigenic (viewed by the body as hostile). (3) They would have to change the recipient's body so it could not or would not make antibodies, the immune system weapons, to expel it.

Only one quite simple situation could answer all three: transplant an organ between identical human twins. With Peter's publication in 1953, Joe and Franny now had the confidence to know *why* a successful kidney transplant could indeed be performed between identical twins. And they were ready to take it on. They just needed the perfect opportunity, the perfect set of twins, one of whom would be dying of renal failure and desperate to borrow a kidney. The other, willing to give it.

Until then, they had to do what they could to help those dying of renal failure, hoping to somehow unveil keys to rejection that could save the lives of those who had no identical donor to offer the ultimate gift.

On October 15, 1954, a physician, Dr. David Miller at the US Public Health Hospital in Brighton, Massachusetts, called the Brigham's transplant team. He said he had a twenty-two-year-old patient, Richard Herrick, recently discharged from the coast guard, who was close to death from Bright's disease. Both of his kidneys were failing catastrophically. Dialysis on the artificial kidney at the Brigham might help.

Joe, of course, was more than interested. But the Brigham physician John Merrill, who was in charge of the artificial kidney, was hesitant. He was reluctant to take on a patient with such a dire disease. He feared dialysis would merely prolong the agonies of death.

Dr. Miller knew there was little chance to change the dialysis team's mind, and, while his first priority was the immediate care of his patient, he also knew that the transplant team might be especially interested in Richard as a transplant candidate. Just before he was about to hang up, he added, "By the way, this patient has an identical twin."

Joe was startled. He was also gratified and excited. For ten years he had been training his hands and fingers to perform the delicate techniques to connect the veins and arteries from a borrowed kidney to those of a host. And now maybe the moment had come.

Allowing no loss of time for either the transplant team to make plans or for the young man whose last chance at life would be in his hands, Joe sent an ambulance to bring young Richard to the Brigham Circle on Huntington Avenue.

PART III

17

Happy Years

WITH A CHARMED LIFE, no curveballs or hiccups to disrupt the smoothness of their childhood, they were living miracles, as much alike as two leaves on a holly bush. Arriving in the world on June 15, 1931, they were what Longfellow called "living poems." With hazel eyes and blond baby fuzz, they were biological wonders: Ronald a little bigger, born first, already wearing a cape of seriousness, while Richard slid into the world with a get-ready grin.

Their parents, Marjorie and Van Buren Herrick Jr., had an older boy, Van, and in four more years would add daughter Virginia. Little did either parent know that they would live only long enough to see their older children into their twenties and Virginia turn twelve. As philosopher William McFee pointed out, "People don't ever seem to realize that doing what's right is no guarantee against misfortune." So, in that enchanting time of their children's early years, Marjorie and Van Herrick knew only joy and how to be good parents, lovers to each other, and grateful troupers in a happy home.

Home was three hundred-plus acres in Rutland, Massachusetts, on the twins' grandfather's dairy farm. He was a retired physician, and his son, the twins' father, was an attorney who preferred farming to practicing law—and no wonder, when the farm was a vista of sweeping golden hayfields that at harvest time smelled like fresh baked bread. Demond Pond, down the hill from the hayfield, would be where the twins would learn to swim and, in winter, to play hockey, where one year Richard sent a puck whizzing, accidentally knocking out part of Ronald's front tooth. Their mother, frantic, rushed him to the local dentist who crowned Ronald's chipped tooth with gold, an unexpected boon as it provided an easy way to tell the twins apart.

First, though, were the early days of life—one parent bouncing a twin on one knee, with the other screaming to be set on the opposite knee. When Richie saw Ronnie sucking a bottle, he, too, wailed for one. Extra hands, arms, legs, and laps always were required to get through those baby years, times two. And, then, when the twins were mobile, they seemed like puppies romping and roaming, with their older brother, Van, assuming sheepdog duties.

As they began riding scooters down the road almost daily to Fay's Country Store, they took on the nickname the *Scooter Twins*. Van, more often than not, was the boss, with serious Ronald his deputy. Ronald never knew *why* exactly, but he always felt responsible for Richard, to be his protector, especially when Richard thought up mischief that Van shot down.

Year-round, their chore of milking the dairy cows was not work but a lark; even cleaning up after them was okay, especially as the cows could be comically named: Dewy, Pewey, Mooey, Stomp-Your-Foot Louie. When the twins were old enough to ride a bike, Van left the house to teach them and came home with bruises and a stare that warned everyone to leave him alone. One Sunday in winter, when their mother was leading them into church, she noticed Richie's pajama bottoms leaking below the hem of his wool pants. Finding their Sunday pants itchy, he and Ronald were wearing their pajamas underneath, but their mother's glimpse of the PJs ended that.

Added to the mystery of their biology was the curious fact that Ron was left-handed, Richie, right. Otherwise, they were so alike that if Ronnie didn't smile to flash his gold, they could mess with anyone's mind. In elementary school, Richie often changed seats with Ronnie just to enjoy their teacher's confusion. Going into a store, Richie would order ice cream, charge it to their grandfather, then go in again to order another. When the clerk remarked that he was just there, he'd angelically reply, "Oh, that was my brother."

MESSING WITH PEOPLE with their duplicate looks was a glorious hobby.

Somewhere along the way, Richie came down with scarlet fever. It was a slight case, and he was the only one in the family to catch it. Soon enough, he was well, and no one thought anything else about it. They were all blissfully unaware that the childhood illness would later raise its ugly head as Bright's disease.

High school sports became their focus: baseball, basketball, hockey. Ronald's left-handedness gifted him an advantage when shooting a basket or sneaking a puck past the goalie. And cars. A day after they got their driver's licenses, they took the family truck for a spin around the farm. After a few laps, they felt that age-old urge to see how fast they could go. With Richie behind the wheel, they zoomed past a hayfield, then unexpectedly saw their father walking out of it. Passing at speeds that rattled the exhaust pipe, they rushed home to pretend nothing had happened. When their father walked in and bluntly said, "Hand over your licenses," Ronald retorted, "But why mine?"

Their father, forever the lawyer, pointed out, "You were an accessory to the crime, and you would have done the same thing if you were driving."

True.

By their senior year of high school, they had grown to five-eight and taken on the habit of folding their arms across their chests when in conversation or intensely concentrating. They had also discovered singing. Or at least what singing could do—in short, mesmerize their listeners. Each alone had a lovely tenor voice, but in duplicate their blended harmonies were stunning. Their duets sounded so unexpectedly angelic, their audiences would wonder if their hearing had been deceived. They sang in church, in school, at town events. Singing got their photos in the paper and gave them a special identity, a way of being known beyond being twins, which they had never had.

Taking the stage, they faced each other, folded their arms across their chests and started with one of their favorites: "I believe for every drop of rain that falls, a flower grows. . . . I believe that somewhere in the darkest night, a candle glows." How beautifully they sang, like a single voice in harmony with itself.

Ah, yes, they had become more than brothers. They were best friends.

In 1948, what being good could not stave off rose up to swallow the family and scar its future. Their mother died. Their father was in poor health. Day by day this new reality took hold. The brothers finished high school. They started college.

Then war, half a world away: on June 25, 1950, seventy-five thousand soldiers from the North Korean People's Army poured across the boundary between the Soviet-backed Democratic People's Republic of Korea and the southern pro-Western Republic of Korea. It was the first military action of the Cold War, threatening World War III.

Ronald Herrick enlisted in the army on November 21. A few weeks later, Richard joined the coast guard.

―――――――

THE BROTHERS NOW WERE APART for the first time. Ronald, as Richard's protector, frequently checked on him. When he learned that Richard had been promoted to second-class petty officer, he took it as a sign that his twin was doing fine. But the war was leaving devastated lives in its wake.

In May 1951, the Herrick children's father died. Called home on emergency leave, the twins had a sad reunion but within days were back to service with a discharge date set for late 1953. Since their little sister, Virginia, now had no parents to care for her, she went to live with family friends. It was Richie who became like a father to her, calling often, writing letters, pulling her close, sharing everyday events.

Their grandfather sold the farm. Their uncle's family invited them to come live with them when they were discharged from the service. And they said yes. A home would be waiting for them in Northborough, Massachusetts. As they served out their terms, Ronald became a sergeant in charge of a radio station in Germany; Richard served on a vessel in the Great Lakes.

In early November 1953, on his discharge, Ronald arrived at his uncle's house. He expected Richard to arrive in a few weeks, but Richard did not show. One morning a letter came. It was from Richard, writing that he was in the Public Health Service Hospital in Chicago. His discharge physical examination had shown that he had high blood pressure, but he assured Ronald that he didn't feel sick, only a little weak. He also said that learning of his medical condition was a complete surprise.

Soon, he wrote again, giving more details. He had been diagnosed with Bright's disease. And he assured Ronald that "he'd lick this thing in a hurry." The twins' grandfather, as a physician, knew how serious Bright's was and gently told Ronald that there was no cure, that the disease would kill Richard.

Alarmed, Ronald packed a suitcase to travel to Richard, but just as he was about to leave, another letter arrived. "Stay put," Richard said. "I'm coming home for Thanksgiving."

But Thanksgiving came, and there was no Richard.

Early in December Ronald received a long letter from Richard's doctor in Chicago. "Your brother is an extremely sick man. He may not live more than two years." He wanted to know what kind of home could be provided for Richard and detailed what Richard would need: a special diet and constant care.

Ronald talked with his Aunt Virginia, and they wrote back assuring they could give Richard all that he would need. In a few days, Ronald got a phone call. It was Richie. "I'm down here at the Brighton Marine Hospital. When can you come over to see me?"

Instantly Ronald drove to Brighton. Richard was so sick, Ronald knew he could not come home. From then, almost every day, Ronald went to the Brighton Hospital to be with Richie. Finally, in May, Richard was allowed to come to his new home for a visit.

As Ronald helped his brother out of the car, he realized how desperately ill Richie was, able only to walk around a little before retreating into the house and taking refuge in bed. But he was upbeat, uncomplaining, and touchingly happy to be out of the hospital and with Ronald. But the seriousness of his condition was impossible to overlook.

Their Aunt Virginia worked hard to prepare Richard's special meals: each day, three slices of salt-free bread, three ounces of meat or fish, a small helping of potato, one egg, green vegetables, and fruit juice. No milk, no ice cream, and no cheating.

In August 1954, Richard began to weaken even more. By October his heart was affected. In the middle of that month, he said he wanted to get back to the hospital. And Ronald dressed him. With every move, Richie nearly collapsed. It seemed that he would not even last to get to the hospital. Finally, Ronald got him downstairs into a chair where Richie rested before laboriously shuffling to the car.

The next days were the saddest and most difficult that Ronald had ever lived, the most stressful he and his brother Van had ever experienced. Their little sister Virginia was full of sorrow. They visited Richard almost every day at Brighton Hospital. Later Ronald would admit, "We knew he wasn't going to make it."

While Ronald sat with Richard, Van, in desperation, talked to Dr. Miller, who was taking care of Richard, and asked if there wasn't something that could be done. Desperately he added, "I'd give him one of my own kidneys if it would help."

Dr. Miller shook his head, saying, "That would be wonderful. But . . . it's been tried a number of times and the donated kidney nearly always degenerates." Then he hesitated. "But wait . . ." He looked at Van, and, as if half thinking aloud and half asking for corroboration, said, "This other brother is a twin, isn't he?"

Realizing that Richard might be a candidate for the Brigham's cutting-edge transplant program, Dr. Miller called the hospital and talked to Dr. John Merrill, head of nephrology. He was hoping that Dr. Merrill would accept Richard for dialysis if not as a transplant candidate, so he mentioned dialysis first. By now Richard was in a partial coma from uremic poisoning. His mental state was deteriorating so rapidly, he appeared psychotic.

For Ronald, seeing his twin wasting away was unbearable. It felt like viewing his own death. When told of Van's conversation with Dr. Miller and the prospects that a transplant between twins might indeed work, Ronald's first thought was, "Of course." Giving part of himself to save his brother felt as immediate and natural as calling Richard's name. Yet on second thought, giving a kidney to his brother felt so much like science fiction, it seemed a gauzy idea, as if shrouded in fog. There were so many questions. Then Dr. Miller's phone call to the Brigham set the prospects of a transplant into motion.

For Ronald, the reality was like being doused with ice water.

His haunting question was: Might they both die?

18

In Terrible Shape

OCTOBER 26, 1954. As Joe waited for the ambulance to bring Richard Herrick to the Brigham, he was excited, apprehensive, and aware of what this case could mean. Here, finally, might be the confluence of all he had learned, the perfect opportunity for a borrowed kidney between identical twins to prove that organs could indeed be successfully transplanted.

Franny was excited and apprehensive as well. As chief of surgery, he was coordinating the essential parts of what might be a historic procedure. He would be the one responsible for any complication, any dropped note, any sidestep or disaster. In a sense, he was the stage manager, and in that role he would not be one to step into the limelight or expect applause. Over all these years, he had been Joe's protector and boss, whom Joe needed to navigate the personalities and ambitions of other players in the transplant field. Now he was about to usher Joe into the role *Joe* had earned.

As soon as Richard arrived, the dialysis machine, built from Dr. Kolff's blueprints, was hooked to an artery and vein in his arm. Dr. Kolff's artificial kidney had been modified by a Brigham surgeon and an engineer to be about five feet long and four feet high, and it was the only chance the poison in Richard's blood could be washed away, the only hope he might regain the strength to withstand surgery.

But when Joe walked into the room to meet this promising case for medical history, his usual optimism sank. Richard was in terrible shape. Usually weighting 150 pounds, he was now down to 98. He was so sick that Joe doubted that Richard could withstand the shock of serious surgery. Furthermore, Richard was so disoriented that Joe wondered what his usual personality was. He wrote in his notes: *When seen on October 27 and 28th, prior to dialysis patient showed… toxic psychosis. Is extremely uncooperative. Behavior erratic and unpredictable. Bit nurse on hand…a psychiatrist called in to evaluate and put such behavior into context.*

Now the questions multiplied. What if Richard *didn't* recover from the toxic psychosis after dialysis? What if the twins were *not* truly identical? What if there was some variation in their chemical similarity that would cause complications and failure?

Relying on his lifelong habits of hard work and sweet stubbornness, Joe organized his plans. He would perform every test in existence to determine if the twins were indeed identical. Decades of research showed that skin grafts between identical twins were accepted with absolutely no rejection. Identical twins' skin exchanges were always accepted as "self." The 1950 case of three boys suspected of being misidentified in the newborn nursery had legally established their identity. And Peter had shown *why*: his groundbreaking discoveries with cattle and mice proved that the privileged time of pre-birth was the *only* time that two individuals could share the life-giving fluids that would ensure they could exchange tissues without rejection.

Even though that research gave Joe confidence, this was the moment to put that finding to work. Transplanting an organ between human twins had never been attempted.

Ready to consult, support, and assist was Franny. Not only did they both know they were on the brink of history, they also knew they were on a downslope of hope. They were risking marring the field of transplantation with another failure.

Franny even thought that if the operation failed, it could set the field of transplantation back a decade or more. On the other hand, if it succeeded it would be "a tremendous shot in the arm" to all of those everywhere working in the field.

Yet, with a patient as sick as Richard, maybe it was not worth the risk.

After six hours of dialysis, things changed. Richard's psychosis disappeared. In three days, he was walking around. Everyone knew that the effect was only temporary. Dialysis could offer Richard only a short-term fix. His only chance for renewed life was receiving a transplant. And the surgery had to be soon.

As the Thanksgiving holiday approached, Richard was allowed to go home.

———

JOE MOVED FORWARD, checking the twins' birth records to see if they had shared a common placenta. Finding that *yes*, they matched the research that Peter had published only a year before in his pre-birth studies, Franny also pointed out that Peter's elegant scientific experiments affected the whole field as nothing before or since, and now they were set to put those discoveries to work in saving Richard. And, in doing so, they would affect the future. For Peter's term *acquired immune tolerance* promised that the future of transplantation could even manage rejection for those who had no twin. Transplanting an organ between those who were unrelated was the holy grail, the answer they were all chasing. Successfully using a cadaver kidney was transplantation's nirvana. Achieving *that* would be more than a moment in history. It would be lasting.

Although Joe and Franny wore the faces of their profession, dispassionate in putting the care of a patient first, no one is born without ego. Borrowing life for Richard would be no small accomplishment for the two men so driven by compassion and the pursuit of excellence. While one was demonstrative, aggressive, and outwardly ambitious, the other so mild that he would flick an insect outside rather than squash it, they were united in this moment of making history. And neither was about to leave the earth without a sign of their existence. Frankly, both were itching to be the first to crack the barrier of transplantation.

BLOOD TESTS ON the twins and their siblings came back proving that their blood groups were identical, yet different from those of their siblings, Virginia and Van. Perfect. Furthermore, the structure and color of Richard and Ronald's eyes were the same. Joe had them come in so he could perform thumb-sized skin grafts between them. Following the research that Franny cited, he put some of their own skin on their forearms, then a patch from the other, so all four skin grafts could be compared. Next, he ordered seventeen formal genetic tests.

Near the Christmas holidays, with Richard well enough to walk around and even visit his home, Joe decided he needed one more test, even though it sounded rather silly. Driven by his need to have—with no lingering questions—all possible proof that Richard and Ronald were indeed chemically similar, he sent them to the Boston police station to be fingerprinted.

It was then that the craziness began.

While this last move seemed a bit over the top, especially since twins' fingerprints seldom match, Joe didn't mind being seen as a

little goofy compared to his need to leave no possibilities for failure. He was feeling the heavy responsibility that in only a few days
he would take a four-inch organ from one healthy body to transplant into another, and there was only one chance for success. No
detail could be set aside.

What did not occur to him was that news reporters hung out
at the police station in hopes of getting a scoop. He was startled
to learn this driving home, when the local news came on the car
radio announcing that Brigham doctors were planning a "daring
operation." He was stunned. The next morning's newspaper head-
lines screamed: TWIN'S LIFE MAY HANG ON FINGERPRINT
TODAY. Suddenly, the scheduled surgery became a world event.

The stakes increased by the minute. In a few days, everyone
would know his name. Joe would be seen as either a hero or a foolhardy gambler.

The press began hanging around the hospital, asking for updates.
The news leak put pressure on everyone. Franny tried to downplay
the preparations as the stakes accelerated for Joe. The reputation of
the hospital was on the line even more than their own careers. Private
failure was a personal sorrow; a public one was branding. There was
no chance now that Ronald and Richard's surgery could be private.
The unspoken sense that a monumental innovation in the universe
of medicine was only days away could not be ignored.

The twins' two sets of fingerprints came back as not alike at all.
By then, though, Joe wasn't really bothered, since all the other tests
showed that they were indeed identical. Another comforting fact was
on the twins' forearms: the button-sized skin exchanged between
them looked as natural as their own. The skin grafts were the most
comforting signal to Joe. They were a reliable prediction that their
kidney tissue would be equally exchangeable, immune to rejection.

For weeks prior to the fingerprint and genetic tests—actually, ever since Richard had been brought to the Brigham as a transplant prospect—the Brigham transplant team had been calling experts in to explore the ethical questions of the surgery. Clergy of all denominations, legal counsel, psychiatrists, various physicians, many with different professional perspectives formed an advisory committee. They agreed that the benefit of a transplant to Richard was obvious, but for Ronald, there would be no physical benefit.

Though unforeseen complications could always occur, removing one of Ronald's kidneys would be low risk. But this pioneering kidney graft was opening up new territory. The Hippocratic oath firmly established the guiding principal for all physicians: to do no harm. Surgeons had been taught to make sick persons well. What would it mean to injure a healthy body by borrowing an organ to give to another? Of course, the organ was not on loan. It was an ultimate gift, a chance for a second life.

The chief of psychiatry monitoring Richard's mental state considered the transplant primarily an ethical problem. He worried most about Ronald. He warned of the pressure being put on him as the donor. "We have to be careful not to be too much swayed by our eagerness to carry out a kidney transplant successfully for the first time. The important question [is] whether as physicians we have the right to put the healthy twin under the pressure of being asked whether he is willing to make this sacrifice."

Because Richard's heart was being affected, the transplant team could not delay its decision. Despite the temporary well-being that dialysis had given him, Richard's condition was perilous, and it was time for a final decision: do the transplant or back off. So the team called Ronald in to discuss all the ramifications of giving one of his kidneys to his dying brother. They went over all the data. They wanted to be able to answer what would surely be Ronald's many questions.

"They were going to cut me open and take out one of my organs. It was shocking even to consider the idea. I felt a real conflict of emotions. Of course I wanted to help my brother, but the only operation I'd ever had before was an appendectomy, and I hadn't much liked that." Ronald's reactions were so very normal, so very human, so relatable to anyone; yet he kept his raw thoughts private.

He was now a freshman at Worcester State Teachers College, studying to be a math teacher. At twenty-three years old, he was young and healthy. He kept ruminating over the most basic, stark facts. Then he decided to talk it over with those he trusted most. Nearly everyone he talked to had the same reaction: a mixture of horror and pity. Horror that a well, strong young man would make such a sacrifice when the outcome was entirely unknown. Pity for the sick brother who was doomed before reaching the prime of his life.

Finally, Ronald went to his Uncle Lee, whose down-to-earth opinions Ronald always respected. Furthermore, his uncle had been the one to generously offer up his home when the twins' parents died. "What would you do?" Ronald asked him.

Uncle Lee was blunt. "Think long and hard about it," plus, "Look at both sides." He then acted out the decision as if he were Ron. "Here's what I'd be thinking. How many people do I know who've had a kidney transplant? None. There aren't any alive. No one could fault me if I didn't do it. The doctors will turn all their attention to Richard. What about me? Are they going to look after me, too? What if I can't make it with just one kidney? And an organ transplant has never worked before. Now instead of one of us dying, we both die? There, you have the negatives."

After a moment of silence, his uncle then pointed out the other side. "The doctors found out that I'm the identical twin because of the skin grafts. Richard's skin on my arm looks better than the piece of my own they transplanted on me. They seem very sure the kidney will take the same way. These doctors know their business. They've done plenty of studying and research. A lot of people get along just fine with only one kidney. If my kidney works for Richard, I'll have saved Richard's life."

After taking another breath, Uncle Lee ended with, "Ronald, I can't tell you what to do. I'm not the one who has to live with the decision. It's *your* decision. You have to decide what's best for both of you."

The whole family was now caught up in Ronald's decision and what it could mean. The excitement of saving Richard's life flowed through the household. Ron was excited at the prospect, yet there was that gnawing fear that it was *his* kidney they were talking about. The chance that his own life would be risked tainted the excitement of trying to save Richard. The grim statistics kept coming back: all other kidney transplants had ended in failure. The only marker that a transplant between himself and Richard could be different was the success of their skin grafts.

Their other genetic tests also pointed to the likelihood that the gifted kidney would escape rejection. Ronald kept touching the grafted patch of skin on his arm, rubbing it, hoping that it might provide a clear-cut answer, and serenity could come with it. Still, the prediction for winning this experiment in biology was only likely, not certain.

A persistent underlying message kept looping in his mind. The square inch of skin borrowed from Richard thriving on this upper left arm was like a badge of twin brotherhood. The two of them were as much alike as biology could make them.

With his Aunt Virginia, Uncle Lee, and brother Van, Ron went into the Brigham to meet with the transplant team. Joe, Franny, and other team members presented the facts as thoroughly and objectively as they could. They discussed preparation for the surgery. They went over the type of anesthesia, the possible complications, and the anticipated result. Joe encouraged Ronald to ask any questions no matter how irrelevant they might seem.

And Ronald had many. Ever the mathematician, he wanted to know the life expectancy of a person with one kidney. He looked at the faces of the transplant team, challenging them. When they admitted they couldn't answer right off, but would find out, Ronald said he'd look forward to coming back to hear it. And the next day, he did. The team followed up with their promise by showing Ronald the actuarial tables from insurance companies. The information showed that there was no increased risk from living with only one kidney. Their statistics revealed that one person in a thousand is either born with a solitary kidney or loses a kidney because of an accident or illness. In those cases, the remaining single kidney enlarged to do the work of two.

"Of course, a person with only one kidney," Joe pointed out, "has to be doubly careful to protect it from damage, because if it were out of commission, he would no longer have a 'spare'." He urged Ronald not to agree to be his brother's donor unless he really wanted to. It was essential for Ronald to be fully aware of the sacrifice and of what it involved.

To be thorough, the transplant team pointed out that the eleven kidney transplants that had already been performed at the Brigham had all failed, but they had involved kidneys from unrelated donors and recipients. The spare kidney had come from a cadaver, from someone who had just died. With Ronald and Richard, the length of time elapsing between the removal and transplant would be minimal. The gifted kidney would be without a blood supply for as short a period as possible. Joe had perfected the surgical techniques to ensure that.

Next, Ronald asked what the chances were that disease would affect his remaining kidney.

The team pointed out that the most critical conditions affecting a single kidney were cancer and trauma. Both were rather rare. Furthermore, the most common types of renal disease affect both kidneys simultaneously.

Weighing most heavily on Joe, Franny, and the other members of the transplant team were the moral and ethical considerations of Ronald's decision. *Yes*, the surgery would be historic, *yes*, this would be a first significant step into the new universe of transplantation, and everyone was excited to take it. But there was also the divergence from usual medical practice in that Dr. Hartwell Harrison would be removing Ronald's healthy kidney, while in contrast, Joe would be performing the transplant on a patient otherwise doomed to die.

At the last meeting, Ronald asked the one question that most rattled him: his future. If he got into trouble, would the hospital provide his health care for the rest of his life? Dr. Harrison was the first to reply, "Of course not," but then immediately added, "Ronald, do you think anyone in this room would ever refuse you care if you needed help?" Joe added that there would be no charges for the surgery and that all those involved in the historic operation would donate their time and skill.

Taking all these facts, Ronald returned home to absorb them. But, of course, he had already quietly made up his mind.

19

"You Get Out of Here and Go Home"

A FEW DAYS BEFORE DECEMBER 20, Ronald Herrick received a phone call. It was the Brigham asking him to come in. The surgery was set for the morning of December 23. The date was the tenth anniversary of Charles Woods's plane crashing on the runway in India. Thinking of that irony, as well as the effect of the scientific phenomenon of Charles's skin grafts lasting beyond the usual, Joe wrote a note on his surgical schedule. *December 23, 1954: kidney transplant.*

Later, he would say, "I was aware of its historical significance. In truth, I treated it as just part of the week's work. Two days prior to the transplant . . . I repaired a double cleft lip, resected a recurrent cancer of the mouth, corrected 'lop' ears in a child, and closed a burn."

While planning the surgery, Joe and Dr. Merrill, the nephrologist on the team, disagreed on whether Richard's diseased native kidneys should be removed. Joe wanted to take both kidneys out immediately, believing that leaving them in could pose a risk of infection that would transmit disease to the new kidney. Dr. Merrill, however, believed that Richard should keep at least one of his native kidneys to act as a sponge, absorbing any harmful substances that might remain. He also felt that if the transplanted kidney failed later on, the native kidney might recover well enough to resume functioning. Joe strongly disagreed.

Franny, after considering both sides, advised Joe to acquiesce. He felt the decision was more in the domain of the medical specialty of urology than of surgery.

With that disagreement solved, the next few days became a countdown. The city of Boston was on edge. The Brigham was primed.

Now Franny, despite his excitement, became cautious. A test run of the surgery on a cadaver might be a wise move. He wanted to make sure the transplanted kidney would fit comfortably in its new site. He and Joe discussed it and agreed to practice the surgery one more time.

Joe had studied and performed the surgery on animal models for years, searching for the right position to place the kidney, the right techniques for securing it and threading the ureter to the bladder in a natural course, or rerouting it. But, still, the idea of a rehearsal on a human body seemed wise.

Joe called pathology departments all across the city asking them to alert him the minute a patient died so he could use the cadaver for a trial run of the transplant. He then concentrated on making his schedule seem normal. He also kept reminding himself that in his lab, he had done the transplant surgery many times, discovering the best techniques by operating on dogs, with their veins and arteries a good match for those of a human. He had been exploring this exact surgery for nearly ten years. In Richard's case, though, he would have no second chance. He added to his notes, "The kidney I was transplanting was the only compatible kidney in the entire universe! I did not want it to fail for any reason—especially for a reason I had neglected to anticipate."

December 20, Ronald reported to the Brigham. Richard was already there, holding onto his life by a disappearing thread. They were put on different floors: Ronald on the first, Richard on the second. During Ronald's discussions with the transplant team, Richard had been too ill to participate. Now that Ronald had been admitted to the hospital and the surgery was scheduled, Richard was distressed to learn of the sacrifice Ronald was about to make. He asked their Uncle Lee what he should do about it.

"Let things stand," his uncle reassured him. "Ronald wants to do it. You'll have the most skillful surgeons; the outcome will then be in God's hands."

At the Murray house that night, Joe and Bobby were throwing a neighborhood holiday party. It was cold and snowy. Seventy-five friends and neighbors were due to arrive at any minute. Joe was making the eggnog. He told his eight-year-old daughter Ginny to stay off the phone. He didn't want to miss the critical phone call that a cadaver was available for the test run. He also worried that Richard would be lost if the surgery were not performed as planned. The dialysis was upsetting the balance of chemicals in Richard's blood, which could cause serious cardiac irregularities. Coordinating the timing of the dialysis with the operation itself could avoid this risk.

When the phone rang, Joe was stirring the eggnog. Yes, a cadaver was available. It was at the Brigham's pathology department.

Joe handed Bobby the eggnog. He kissed her goodbye and rushed to his car.

Anxiously he drove the icy roads into the city. And with his left-handed surgical instruments met Franny in the postmortem room. Together, they went through the entire operation, thinking of every possible surgical mishap. The test run took a couple of hours.

By the time Joe made it back home, the last of the guests were leaving. He drank some eggnog with them. And soon after he went to bed, feeling prepared to do the historic surgery three days later.

———

THE NIGHT OF DECEMBER 22, Richard sent Ronald a message: "You get out of here and go home!"

Ronald sent back: "I am here and I'm going to stay here. And that's it."

In the Murray home, Bobby told her children, "Daddy's doing an important operation tomorrow. Let's pray and hope it goes well." They knelt, and Bobby led them in prayer. Even though they often did so, that night the prayer felt very different.

At dawn the next morning, Joe drove Route 9 to the Brigham, waving to commuters as he usually did. Suddenly, the car radio carried a news report of the historic surgery to be performed that day. Joe was still not prepared for the media attention. He also realized "it was both an education and a shock to discover how sustained and widespread public interest in organ transplantation was." He knew that while some hoped for a success, others had taken the time to warn him that he could be jeopardizing his career by performing the risky surgery. In any case, if not all the radios in the world were tuned in to hearing what he and the Brigham were about to do, certainly most in the cars of his fellow commuters were.

As the stress built up, he took comfort in knowing that he had done all he could to be prepared for this moment. He also concentrated on the advice of a favorite theologian, Thomas Merton, who said that one's work should be a "wordless prayer."

Two days before Christmas, a Thursday, both Richard and Ronald were under anesthetic—Richard with a spinal, but sedated and unable to urge Ronald to go home. Joe walked into one operating room. Another surgical team with Franny and Dr. Harrison were in an adjacent room.

The surgery was set to begin on Richard at 8:45 a.m. By 9:50, the blood vessels to Ronald's kidney were isolated and exposed, but still attached. Joe took a deep breath and gave Dr. Harrison the go-ahead to sever the blood supply from Ronald's left normal kidney.

From that moment, the timing was critical. In a moment of near catastrophe, the clamp that Dr. Harrison had put on Ronald's aorta suddenly slipped. A whoosh of blood flooded the operative field. Jumping into emergency mode, the surgical team offered hands to help control the bleeding. As soon as Dr. Harrison repaired the artery, he lifted out the donated kidney.

Wrapping it in a cold, wet towel, a member of the team then set it in a sterile stainless-steel basin and handed it to Franny. Quickly, but gently, Franny walked the gifted kidney to the adjacent room where Joe picked it up and placed it into the "bed" he had prepared for it in Richard's abdomen. Now he worked rapidly to reestablish blood flow. He began suturing artery to artery, vein to vein, much as Carrel had taught fifty years before.

Clamps on two of Richard's arteries, one supplying blood to his kidney, another to his leg, held back the means to keep the borrowed tissue alive. At 10:10, Joe finished joining arteries to the gifted kidney. The veins were taking longer. All the while, Joe was aware of the time ticking away—everyone was—but he could only continue to work carefully and systematically. At 11:15, he pulled through the last stitch.

Soon now, they would all know if he had succeeded.

A collective hush hung over the room as he gently removed the clamps from the vessels attached to Ronald's transplanted kidney. For a total of an hour and twenty-two minutes, it had been without blood flow. Everyone on the team was breathing shallowly, barely pulling in air, as they watched Richard's new kidney suddenly turn pink. Smiles broke out behind their masks, the creases at their eyes the outward signs of joy and relief.

Ten minutes later, Joe removed the last clamp from Richard's iliac artery, and immediately the pulse in Richard's right foot began visibly thumping.

The transplanted kidney lay comfortably in its new site, pulsing with life-giving fresh blood. Next, urine visibly began flowing from the catheter inserted in it. Joe soon began rerouting it into the bladder in its natural way. But until then, urine flowed so vigorously, it had to be mopped up from the floor. Comically, gloriously, the essential fluid spurted, making puddles, no longer stymied by disease.

———————

NEWS OF THE SUCCESSFUL transplant sped around the world. Within days, those who were studying renal failure knew of it. Franny pointed out that the discovery of ether 108 years before had taken months to be known. And now, even science, with its age-old methods bound to facts and truth, was being affected by modern communication.

The next step was to duplicate the success of the transplant to prove that the procedure would indeed be lasting.

To many in the world of traditional medicine, the transplant's success seemed a fluke. Doubters pointed out that many coincidences had to be in place to match its success. The gem at the center of the sparkling achievement was that the transplant had been performed on identical twins. And those twins had been young. One had been in the end stage of renal failure and also in the hands of a physician who referred the case to a transplant surgeon and team. Not everyone could be so lucky.

Joe and Franny and the Brigham team did not yet feel justified in publishing their results. Their scientific achievement had to be duplicated by others. Besides, to really make the surgery a success, Richard had to live. And Ronald had to show that giving away an organ did not compromise his future.

To Ronald and Richard the Socratic discussions were of little consequence. Their lives were what mattered. They were more than relieved. They were in shock with joy.

And so was Franny. He noted that since the Brigham team had overcome the immune barrier by transplanting a kidney between identical twins, it had proven that tissue transplantation was here to stay. More than likely, too, adding to his and the hospital staff's euphoria were the rumors being whispered in the halls: Richard was falling in love.

———

ON JANUARY 29, 1955, Joe wrote: *Since operation five weeks ago, Richard has done very well. The wounds healed rapidly, his transplant has functioned immediately and continuously. The course of the future is unknown and the best method of future treatment is a matter of conjecture only. In my opinion, his future longevity depends entirely on his transplant as an "all or none" phenomenon. Either the transplant will take or it will not. Therefore every possible and theoretical mode of protecting this transplant should be taken as soon as possible.*

During those five weeks, Richard not only awoke to a second life, he began to luxuriate in it. Almost from the moment he shook off the sedation of surgery, his eyes took in the sight of Clare Burta, a nurse from Glace Bay, Nova Scotia, who was too far away to go home for that Christmas holiday. And since she couldn't go home, she was on duty in the recovery room, where she first saw Richard. And he, her—each looking at the other with the same infatuated wonder.

Slim, with a light complexion, dark brown eyes, a reluctance to ever stop moving, and a dry sense of humor, Clare seemed to have a witty remark for every other moment. On that first day in the recovery room, she noted, "Most of the patients I see are unconscious, but Richard wasn't because he had a spinal. It was just four days later on December 27 that I was sent up on private duty in the room where Richard was, and I spent the whole day with him. That did it."

She not only attended to Richard's every need, she also kept him aware of reconnecting with life. When Richard wondered if he shouldn't laugh so often for fear of breaking open his stitches, she quipped, "Of course you should. It's good for you."

Not until April would they have their first date. After all, other matters had to be attended to first, such as getting Richard home as well as seeing about his two diseased kidneys still in place. For a while, Richard was the only person on earth walking around with three kidneys.

As for Joe, he felt that the Herrick operation was "no different from any of the other procedures that surrounded it." Or at least he pretended that. On Christmas Day, he was at the Newton-Wellesley Hospital emergency room suturing a cut on a child's forehead.

Ronald went home the first week in January and picked up where he left off in his college classes. Richard, in the Brigham, began eating all the foods he'd been denied before and spent the days flirting with Clare. On January 19, only twenty-seven days after the historic operation, he was discharged, and Ronald went to the hospital to accompany him back to a full life.

They were now household names. Almost everyone in America knew of the Herrick twins. As they reached the hospital door, the press was waiting. Flashbulbs popped. Writers gathered around for interviews. Ron, always ready to hide his feelings, said he hadn't been anxious before the surgery at all. He deferred credit to the doctors, "We felt very strongly that it would work. Of course, it hadn't been done before. But they knew their research."

Back home in Northborough, Richard took up what he had been unable to do for nearly a year, eating everything in sight, taking walks outside, even thinking about going to college. Before the surgery, his heart had been enlarged and there had been fluid in his lungs. All that disappeared. Being alive was a shock, a welcome one; he realized he now had a future. He began thinking mostly of Clare.

After a few weeks, when his blood pressure began to rise and signs of infection surfaced, Joe scheduled surgeries to remove Richard's diseased kidneys. Joe and Dr. Merrill now agreed that the transplanted kidney was working so well, it was reasonable to remove the nonfunctioning ones.

On March 29, Joe took out the first one; the other surgery was scheduled for June. In April, Richard took Clare out in his new car to, as he said, see how it ran. They drove around. Clare would soon say, "I knew then I wanted to marry Richard, and I kind of guessed he felt the same about me, but he hadn't said anything." Richard would later admit that he'd already decided the whole thing by that time. But he was still getting used to a retrieved life and didn't want to jinx it.

To make sure that her feelings were what she thought they were, Clare took a job in a hospital in Texas. She stayed there for three months in the midst of oil-well country until a proposal from Richard arrived in the mail. It was "on Friday the thirteenth of all things," Clare said, laughing, and "we decided to get married in Texas. . . . We knew there'd be a lot of to-do in Massachusetts where everyone knew about Richard . . . and marriage to me is a serious thing." She had the quiet, simple ceremony she'd always wanted.

20

"Freedom from Burden"

THE HISTORIC SURGERY on Richard Herrick—the culmination of Joe's expertise, Franny's guidance, Peter's research, and the diligence of the transplant team at the Brigham—would prove not to be a fluke. Over the next four years, a further seven transplants were performed between identical twins at the Brigham, and while not all of those were as successful as that between Ronald and Richard, the surgery changed medicine. By the autumn of 1963, thirty twin transplants had been performed throughout the world. Of the twins who were women, several had successfully given birth, perhaps the harshest test of nature to a human body, and certainly the ultimate workout for a kidney.

Now the focus was on what Joe called the "holy grail"—a successful transplant not just between identical twins but between unrelated donors and hosts. Not until then could it be said that the world of medicine had created another man-made miracle, retrieving a number of humans from heartrending suffering or looming death.

The thorny problem of compatibility remained.

Scientists and doctors had flirted with the idea of borrowing health from one to strengthen another—or even to save a life—for hundreds of years. In 1818, an English obstetrician gave blood from several donors to women dying of postpartum hemorrhage. He had practiced on dogs, using a funnel and pump that worked with gravity, but of course technique was not the issue. Not until blood groups were discovered could blood be transfused to save a life. Until then, blood transfusion theory was as valid as the belief that the earth was flat.

Likewise, as the transplant world moved from the special situation of surgery between identical twins to borrowing organs from unrelated donors, it grappled with *how* to manufacture a perfect compatibility to escape rejection. Of course, Peter had found the solution years before. After discovering that cows producing twins interchanged cells between the calves before birth, he learned to duplicate the phenomenon. He followed the formula and exchanged cells between two unrelated mice and also unrelated chickens while they were in the womb. That was all right for mice and chickens, but it was completely unrealistic for the human world. An artificial means had to be found.

Today, it is difficult to realize how little was known about the immune system before World War II. Physicians and scientists had always been aware of something important in the way the human body responded to viruses and bacteria. *Freedom from burden*, the literal meaning of *immunity*, was recognized as a kind of symphony of biology. But no one understood its parts. As Joe, Franny, and Peter pushed themselves to learn how to manipulate that biology, they knew they were in the presence of perfection. Sixty years later, when Oxford mathematician Marcus du Sautoy said that understanding the human body "[is] something so complex that it makes quantum physics look like a high school exercise," he captured perfectly the challenge facing Joe, Franny, and Peter as they tried to expand transplantation's success in the 1950s.

Attacking the problem of incompatibility on a cellular level made the most sense. In his lectures, Franny liked to point out that every cell in the body is a complete factory, and this factory's purpose is to keep the body well. He liked to illustrate the size of the red and white blood cells that play leading roles in immunity and maintaining health. We can imagine him standing in a lecture hall gleefully drawing a letter "o" on a blackboard, saying, "If a line of red blood cells were arranged side by side, like coins in a collection, or a row of checkers awaiting play on a checkerboard, there would be room for about 150 [human red blood cells] across this round hole of the letter 'o'." Then, in explaining some basic principles in the immune system, he would add: "Some of the white cells in the blood, such as the small lymphocytes [which are the cells that make the weapons to attack a foreign tissue in the body, such as a transplanted kidney], are slightly smaller, about 3.5 micra in diameter." Up to 200 of these could fit side by side in the middle of the printed letter "o." Putting this in context, he liked to add that the total mass of someone's cells weighs about fifty-five pounds in an adult. The rest of the body consists of connective tissues, bones, and body fluids outside of cells. This simple explanation of the architecture of a patient's body helped explain how Franny and the transplant team had to think at a cellular level while caring for a transplant patient.

Franny compared the immune system to a fort. From the moment of birth, each life, through the weapons of its immune system, is protected, defended, and given the best chance for survival in a world that is not always hospitable. In each lifetime a few serious infections come along to give the immune system an exhausting workout. In a world teeming with bacteria, a body's structures and processes watch over each life, defending the portals of entry, such as skin, which is the first line of defense, not only for holding in fluids, but also for blocking out invaders in the environment. Tears wash out intruders and can even kill entering germs. Saliva washes out germs that breech the mouth, another portal of entry, and even has the means to kill them if they cling to interior tissue. While the gut takes in foreign substances for nutrition, it also sorts out those that are harmful and then kills or expels them. This symphony of biology exists in all higher forms of life, and perhaps the most magical and impressive act of the immune system is its ability to identify those bacterial and viral diseases it has met before, fought, and defeated. From each encounter, the system builds immunity to that invader, recognizing it when it tries or succeeds in breeching the portals again.

Early on, immune system memory caught the attention of physicians as they observed how Europeans, who had built immunity to certain diseases over centuries, tragically infected the peoples they colonized. Native Americans, for example, had no weapons to battle the viruses and bacteria brought from Europe, and often perished. The body's ability to remember the first exposure to a virus or bacteria days, weeks, months, or years later became a major factor in developing lifetime vaccines to resist deadly diseases. And learning how to trick cellular memory would soon become a major turning point in the science of transplanting an organ.

Searching for a strategy to manipulate this system of defense, Joe, Franny, Peter, and the transplant team focused first on the two-part weapon system that the immune system creates: antigens and antibodies. Literally meaning "the thing that generates antagonism," an *antigen* calls forth the body's most powerful weapon, an *antibody*. When the antigen gains entry into the body, it sets off an alarm, arousing an immune response that prompts specific antagonists. These antibodies in the blood inactivate the invading antigen and make it ready for removal. The battle between antigens and antibodies is apparent when a body spikes a fever, a signal of the warfare going on.

In his lectures on the immune system, Franny liked to use lobar pneumonia as a common example of a war within a body. He especially liked this as an example because it is an illness often represented in films and novels with dramatic effect: a character lies deathly ill, then, over the course of a few hours, the fever falls; the person sweats profusely and becomes well. On the other hand, depending on the story's plot, the antigens win the battle; bacteria overwhelm the defenses; the character dies. The result in real life is shattering grief. In fiction, the imaginary experience is always a sobering and stunning example of the immune system's power.

Searching for a method to trick the immune system into accepting a donor's kidney, the transplant team embraced Peter's research that showed a body could be manipulated to *tolerate* a borrowed organ. Backing up that principle was the fact that some viruses normally stay present in the human body without being attacked and without causing any disease at all.

Hoping to duplicate that same acceptance for a borrowed organ, the transplant team considered several possibilities. One was to introduce cells from a donor as a decoy to build immunity to a kidney transplanted from that exact donor later. Peter suggested paralyzing the immune system with repeated skin grafts, convincing the immune system to more or less give up attacking the invader. The transplant team even considered removing the thymus, which revs up the immune system soon after birth, and/ or the spleen, which is an active home for producing antibodies. After considering many strategies, Joe, Franny, and Peter eventually settled on what World War II had revealed: that survivors of the nuclear blasts in Japan had weakened immune systems. And so, to duplicate that finding, they decided to try whole-body irradiation using X-ray beams.

Joe found information from research, performed years before but not fully understood at that time, to add to their plan. It gave hope that the cellular response in a transplant patient could be changed to make it a welcoming host for a borrowed kidney.

Dr. John Mannick and E. Donnall "Don" Thomas had been working in Cooperstown, New York. A hematologist, Thomas had been trained at the Brigham, developing the stunning idea of matching the immune systems of two separate unrelated individuals by using bone marrow cells. Bone marrow, manufactured in the bones, produces both red and white blood cells. White blood cells, which produce antibodies, are the ones to attack an invading antigen, such as a transplanted kidney.

Thomas's approach was to harvest some of the patient's bone marrow cells, store them under conditions that would keep them alive for a time, then, after a patient's whole body was irradiated to wipe out the remaining bone marrow cells, transplant the kidney, *and then* put the stored marrow cells back in. Next, these would multiply—hopefully—to build back a functioning immune system with no desire to attack a transplanted organ—at least not as vigorously as if it had not been manipulated. Furthermore, the transplanted organ would be given a grace period before the host's body could launch an attack against it. That was the thinking, and that was the hope.

Eventually, Joe and Franny would alter this strategy by giving bone marrow cells from the donor, thinking these would engineer a more welcoming host for a donor's kidney.

Now the Brigham transplant team had their protocol. In 1957, they began a study of total-body irradiation on twelve kidney transplant patients. Transplant candidates would be placed in front of an X-ray machine with the beam focused on their whole body to produce what was to be called *whole-body irradiation* to suppress the patients' immune defenses. The donor's bone marrow cells were then injected, with the aim that the patient would recognize the donated kidney as "self." Follow up with the surgery: put in the borrowed kidney.

It was a trick that Franny liked to describe as a "beachhead" approach: bombard with irradiation, "then have a shore party of bone marrow cells to prepare the way for the main invasion by a borrowed kidney."

But battering a dying patient's immune system with whole-body irradiation would turn out to be trickier than anyone thought. Manipulating the body's exquisite power without destroying it would not come easily or quickly. And certainly not as smoothly as Joe, Franny, Peter, and the transplant universe hoped.

The euphoria of Ronald and Richard's successful transplant was quickly becoming short-lived, rimmed with the nightmare darkness of not being able to expand it beyond the safety of the compatible immune systems of identical twins. Death would haunt the renal-transplant unit at the Brigham. And Joe, Franny, and Peter would be wrapped in the grim reality that biology would not give up its secrets without harsh, heartrending failures.

As Thomas Starzl, who would become a renowned transplant surgeon at the University of Pittsburgh, said, this time brought "a long list of tragic failures leavening the occasional encouraging notions such as those in identical twins." Caring for one of those twelve, Gladys Loman, a thirty-one-year-old mother of two, would break Joe.

21

"Oh, Dear, Haven't
You Heard?"

JEAN MEDAWAR SUFFERED her own personal crisis in the middle of the fifties. It was not physical, but one of the soul, which in its own way can be just as debilitating.

In short, she wanted a life of meaning of her own. She didn't want to be defined simply as being Peter's wife.

In 1953, she bought her first diary, thinking its publication might one day be a great literary event. But when she saw the pages filled with her children's dental appointments, the days she nursed their cases of mumps, the times noted for school plays or the opera, and never a journal about her feelings, she changed her mind. Obviously, she was not producing a literary masterpiece but a work that would bore the eyeballs out of anyone.

She recognized she tried too hard to be both mother and father, to make up for the time that Peter couldn't give to fatherhood. She began to long for a goal, for some skill that would set her apart. She went over her early aspirations and recalled a strange and naive dream that as a forty-year-old woman made her laugh. At the outbreak of the war, she had daydreamed that if she could only meet Hitler, she could get him to see that there was no such thing as *race*, only the human race. And now, likewise, in the early years of the Cold War, she decided that if she could only speak Russian, she could help Russians realize their folly in fearing the West.

She signed up for evening classes in Russian. When she heard that Russian visitors had arrived at Peter's lab, she rushed to greet them. Gushing Russian phrases to make them feel welcome, she then listened to them respond in a torrent of Russian, none of which she understood.

But then, when the Soviet Academy of Sciences invited Peter to lecture at the University of Moscow in December of 1955 and included her in the invitation, she pulled out her Russian books and went at it again.

Getting off the plane with Peter, she was struck by ice-cold air that made it hard to breathe and prompted her to exclaim, "It was so cold that I thought the fluid in my eyes would freeze. And everything looked grey or black. . . . Formless women swaddled against the cold wielded shovels to keep the December streets clear of snow."

At Peter's lecture, she sat next to an entomologist and exchanged Russian phrases with him until Peter started lecturing. Since Peter's every sentence was translated, his usual dramatic lecturing was squeezed to a trickle. One sentence, then another, until soon his lecture became so drawn out that Jean became proof of what Peter claimed, "that there was no sleep so refreshing as that induced by the voice of a lecturer in the dark." Furthermore, Peter joked that before he learned to leave the lectern and walk about to engage his listeners, "putting them to sleep was one of the greatest blessings that lay in his power to bestow."

Bestow he did, and generously. As Jean slid sideways into the entomologist, using him as a pillow, every once in a while she jerked awake to see that Peter was still at it.

Back home in London, she gave up her self-appointed Russian-language goals and called a family planning clinic, offering to volunteer. She noted in her diary that her days spent at the clinic opened her eyes to "how many people spent their lives in a state of quiet despair." And as might be expected, she soon ascended to the top of the clinic's administration and then to the organization's national level.

Peter's career flourished. He was flying around to give lectures in America and Europe. Having her own commitments, Jean now rarely went with him. She always had time, though, to help ease his workload, marveling at the obsessive level with which he always went at his work. He answered letters in twenty-four hours, laid out his next day's clothes before going to bed, never relaxed before a meal with a glass of wine, ate too fast, smoked too much, and never slept well. Once she teased him into promising that he would not work one evening a week.

He assured her that he was different, that he didn't need rest because a lot of his work was "as good as a rest." His favorite description to explain who he was rested on the word *obsessional.* He said that a fellow obsessional could recognize the danger sign of being one when you saw "the tendency to regard the happiest moments of your life as those that occur when someone who has an appointment to see you is prevented from coming."

He never slept late and on weekends woke Jean by standing near her bed with a slice of bread and honey and large cup of what he called "wake-you-uppo-tea."

His gifts to her were expressions not only of his love but of his recognition of how much she gave to him. When parking meters were common, he gave her a boxful of coins to feed them. On her birthday and Christmas, he asked her to go out and buy whatever she liked. When she playfully retorted, "I expect you'd like me to wrap it up," he laughed and instructed, "and don't forget to write on the tab: *To my darling wife from her devoted husband.*"

Later, Jean would torment herself with wishing she had not played that game. It might have been better for his health to have him do easy, ordinary chores, but she got pleasure from thinking she was saving him for Higher Things. Once he said, "I want to load you with jewels." And she let him.

In the early spring of 1960, they went to Boston for Peter to give the Dunham Lectures at Harvard Medical School. Inspired by putting her to sleep in Moscow, Peter spent two years engineering a remedy for soporific lecturing. And he had a flair for the dramatic to draw from. Now he was ready to pull out his new style. He wanted to present the whole story of immunological tolerance and its implication in a conversational way. He aimed for everyone to be able to understand him, not just scientists and physicians. He wanted to open the world to comprehending the symphony of biology, to the exquisite precision of how the human body protects itself against an invasion of disease. He wrote out his lecture and then condensed it into notes with key words as reminders. He timed each hour's talk to the minute.

The day of his lecture at Harvard Medical School, crowds of faculty, scientists, physicians, and guests headed to the largest amphitheater. Soon it was not large enough. Opening up other amphitheaters, staff set up loudspeakers to carry Peter's voice, and the overflow crowd rushed in.

As Franny arrived at the lecture hall, he noted how the air buzzed with excitement. "The intensity of scientific interest in a rapidly growing field is something few can appreciate unless they witness it." He predicted that Peter's discoveries were so valuable to the future well-being of mankind that his contribution to science would soon catch the attention of the Nobel Foundation in Sweden. He declared that the new field of immunology was hot, rapidly growing, and attracting scientists worldwide. Peter was known now as the father of immunology, and he was constantly in demand.

As Jean sat in the audience, she saw how Peter had perfected his new take on giving a lecture. He left the lectern and walked up and down. He seemed "as though supercharged and unable to be still." Everyone in the audience felt that he was speaking directly to them. He was that engaging, that personal. And, of course, the information was so compelling that everyone felt privileged to be at this pivotal moment of a historical scientific revolution.

Word spread. The scientific world embraced him as a genius. The invitations began pouring in. That September, Milan Hašek invited Peter to speak at a meeting in Czechoslovakia. This was the colleague whose investigative studies on chickens had duplicated and run parallel to Peter's own studies of pre-birth acquired tolerance, and Hašek was eager to meet Peter in person. It was known that he had a personality as vivacious as Peter's, which would give Jean the prospect of witnessing the fireworks of unleashed energy and rare intellect of two unique men. She was eager to go and began packing right away.

She and Peter decided to drive there and ordered a car to be picked up at a factory outside of Hamburg. When they arrived from London, the car was waiting, and Jean did much of the driving, heading first to a lovely river hotel, then to Vienna. Stopping there to have dinner, they watched two old Charlie Chaplin films, during which Peter laughed so much that people in the seats around them laughed as much at him as at Charlie.

Hašek's reputation as an innovative, fearless scientist was already generating talk that he would be considered for a Nobel Prize. At the time, no one suspected that in eight years, the Soviet Union would invade Czechoslovakia and revise Hašek's science to fit the communist government's ideological needs. In September 1960, oblivious to that danger to science, Peter and Jean eagerly drove in their new car toward the arranged meeting with the esteemed scientist.

Reaching the Czech border, they found it guarded with a high wire fence. Peter remarked that it sloped inward and down, clearly not to prevent people entering the country but to keep those inside from leaving. And Jean noted that guards searched the car as though they would be pleased to find stolen goods.

Dr. Hašek was waiting for them at their hotel. And the threatening atmosphere lifted. His effusive personality showered them like confetti. After years of following each other's careers, their delight in finally meeting was contagious. Over the next few days, as Hašek and Peter visited colleagues, discussing the latest results from experiments, the excitement of the new understanding of the mechanics of immunology took on a party-like air. There was joy in the new science being revealed and embraced. Taking long walks up local mountains, sharing dinners in lovely settings, the talk never ceased. Multiple toasts were made "to England," "to your country!" "to peace," "to friendship," and on and on, punctuated with laughter, added to and repeated, until there was barely time left to drink wine.

On the last day of their visit, Hašek drove Jean and Peter to Prague for a party at his house. The light was fading, and the road was hard to see. He turned sharply to the right off a main road just as Peter asked, "What does that notice say?" Jean, sitting behind them, read, *Danger, no entry—road up*. The next moment the car's front wheels hit something hard, and it bounced off to crash into something else. The engine quit; the car tilted to the right, hanging by its tires over a six-foot trench.

When they all sat up, Jean saw Peter's face running with blood from a cut on his forehead. The side of her own face was beginning to swell. She managed to get out of the car to check Peter's cut. Finding that it was not deep and that he was not seriously hurt, she turned to see Dr. Hašek standing by the car in a state of shock, repeating over and over, "What have I done? I should have seen that notice. I may have damaged Peter's brain."

Hugging him, Jean said not to worry; they both were all right, and she humorously affirmed that Peter's brain was still in place. A bystander called an ambulance. By the time it arrived, a man who had come to look at the wreck also fell into the trench. He got so banged up that when the ambulance finally came, he got in, too, which became a story that Peter loved to tell over and over.

On their drive home the next day, as Peter and Jean stopped at the Czech border, no one remarked on their obvious injuries. Peter said, "They're not surprised. They just think we've been beaten up."

A month after their trip, the phone rang in their house in London. Jean answered to hear her close friend Marghanita Laski's voice saying in an excited tone, over and over, "Congratulations, congratulations!"

"What for?"

"Oh, dear, haven't you heard? I don't think I should be the first to tell you." But Marghanita blurted the news: Peter had won the Nobel Prize in Medicine.

In a matter of days, Peter and Jean were on their way to Stockholm. Peter was only forty-five, a ridiculously young age to have achieved a contribution significant enough to impress the Nobel committee. As expressed in Alfred Nobel's will, which set up the funds and administration for the prize, the awards should be given to "those who shall have conferred the greatest benefit to mankind." And, certainly, that qualified Peter in the field of medicine.

His studies of acquired immune tolerance were the foundation for understanding how Richard Herrick could accept Ronald's gifted kidney without rejecting it. The surgery could have been successful with only the decades-old study that identical twins' skin could be exchanged with perfect acceptance, but understanding *how* identical twins became a perfect tissue match gave the assurance that organ transplantation was indeed possible as a shift in the treatment of disease. And, it promised that from understanding the biological process, a boundless future lay ahead.

———————

As THE DECADE turned from the fifties to the sixties, life seemed golden. An armistice signed in July 1953 brought an end to fighting in Korea. A new war opened on an intellectual front that could be called by no other name than *cold*, as two world powers with fundamental disagreements "over human rights, individual liberties, [sparred] over the direction of history and the destiny of man." As Arthur Schlesinger Jr. would say fifty years later in a Pulitzer Prize-winning memoir, "New generations may well wonder what all the shouting was about." There was the threat of nuclear war, yes, but somehow peace between nations held.

This transition from one decade to the next was also a tough time for Joe and Franny. Beginning in 1957, there were seven years of nightmarish failure as they sought to turn the Herrick transplant into a miracle that could benefit all people, not just identical twins. And though, for Peter, there would always be the satisfaction that the 1960 Nobel Prize Committee had recognized the irreplaceable importance of his work, it would not be long before he entered his own nightmare of losing the use of most of his body, leading to his frequent comment, "I have a very decided preference to stay alive."

22

Chasing the Holy Grail

By 1958, MORE AND MORE Americans were buying a house, getting an education, and starting families with many children, and a new expression began peppering their speech. "Romance was 'the love bit,' Metrecal 'the diet bit,' and Alfred Hitchcock's *Psycho* 'the thrill bit'." There were even surgeons doing "the transplant bit," such as Thomas Starzl in Pittsburgh, Joe Murray in Boston, and John Mannick in Cooperstown, New York.

Chasing the holy grail of transplanting a kidney from a donor unrelated to the host was failing miserably. In the late fifties, Joe had scientists visit for two or three days at a time, staying in his home to go to his transplant lab. Peter stayed in ten-year-old Ginny's room. So did Milan Hašek, filling the house with what Joe called "his hearty, friendly" personality. Ginny recalls Peter being so large it was as if the walls stretched to fit him in.

At the hospital, Joe never took the elevator but climbed the stairs to stay fit. He and Bobby played tennis at least once a week, sharpening Bobby's reputation as a fierce competitor. When she and Joe won tournaments in mixed-double matches, Joe made a habit of pouring Raisin Bran and chocolate into their trophies. Eating his strange concoction from their winning cup was the best use for it, he said.

Still a "cockeyed optimist," he insisted to his six children that difficulties were opportunities. In his nonconfrontational way, he was stern in his demand that they meet his standards. He allowed only one phone in the house and made all the kids stay off it when he was waiting for a donor kidney to be available.

There was no yard help; the kids did it. They washed the storm windows and stored them away. As their family grew, their houses became bigger. A TV set was finally allowed to be brought into the den in 1958. But the viewing time was set to just an hour a week.

Bobby exercised her music muscles by performing in local operas. Exerting her aspirations to be known not only in Joe's shadow, she wrote a musical for the local Junior League titled *Jackie and the Cornstalk*, which had a literacy theme: Jackie climbed up the cornstalk for reading lessons.

Joe continued to leave the house every morning in the dark and, as the sun came up, waved to his fellow commuters on Route 9 driving into Boston. And his love for Bobby never waned. He was a romantic at heart, dipping into the habits of his youth, often courting her as if on a first date.

————

In 1957, the Brigham transplant team began their study of twelve kidney transplants between those who were not genetically identical. Their strategy of preparing the patients for a transplant using total-body irradiation followed by bone marrow transfusion was now put in place. In Joe's lab, studies with dogs did not lead him to think the approach would be successful, but his studies with rabbits and mice were moderately encouraging. So the combination of irradiation and bone marrow infusions seemed, at the time, the most promising for those patients doomed to die.

Of the twelve in need of new kidneys, disease was not the only cause of their troubles. Gladys Loman, a thirty-one-year-old mother of two with a very rare physical condition, would leave a mark on medical history, and on Joe. In what seemed a case of appendicitis, she was rushed to an outlying hospital for surgery.

When the surgeon removed the infected mass, he was startled to see it was not her appendix he was holding, but her kidney. Even worse, Gladys was found to be one of those rare people who had been born with only one. Knowing of the Herrick twins' successful surgery and the transplant program at the Brigham, the surgeon immediately called Joe. Joe knew that the only chance to save Gladys was to give her a kidney. And it had to be done right away. He went to his good friend and fellow surgeon Don Matson.

As Joe asked Don for a spare kidney for Gladys, Don jokingly commented that he had been involved in one Nobel Prize venture, and now perhaps he'd become involved in another!

Immediately, Joe and Franny arranged for Gladys to come into the Brigham for a transplant. Before she arrived, she was given dialysis, which improved her health tremendously. In a few days she was up and about, leading a normal life within the hospital, though there was no "normal" for her to return to. Time was short. There was no other way to solve her problem than to borrow the child-sized kidney that Don Matson, as a pediatric neurosurgeon, had to sacrifice in an operation he had performed on one of his pediatric patients suffering from hydrocephalus. Inserting a shunt to drain the brain fluid out through the child's bladder meant that one kidney, healthy and of no longer use to the child, could be given to Joe.

The decision to try to save Gladys by controlling rejection using whole-body irradiation followed by bone marrow transfusions was a difficult one. Joe, Franny, and the transplant team consulted members of the surgical service—physicians, pathologists, radiologists, scientists from the medical school, and neighboring hospitals. No one had ever received the treatment that the transplant team outlined for her.

As the team gave high doses of total-body irradiation to Gladys, she lay on a stretcher about nineteen feet from the irradiation portal, so she was fully exposed to the X-ray beams. The goal was to suppress antibody-producing cells from the system that produced them in the spleen, lymph nodes, and bone marrow. Her body would then be prepared to receive the kidney with no weapons ready to reject it.

Franny and Joe hoped the precise dose was right; they needed her antibody defenses against bacteria not to be depressed too much. They sought to achieve the balance of survival. And that balance was fragile.

Since her defenses against infection would be lowered to a dangerous level, they had to keep her away from bacteria. The safest place was the operating room. After her first irradiation session, she moved in, ready to live there for a month or more to sustain her borrowed kidney when it was transplanted and protect it against rejection. In that sense, she would be like a victim of nuclear war, and there were no lessons to draw on. No one knew what to expect.

Anyone who went in to see her had to have a complete change of clothes. They wore a cap, a mask, and, after a scrub of the hands, sterile gloves. So Gladys lived, passing the hours in the only way she could survive.

Soon after the course of irradiation was complete, she was given thirty-six billion marrow cells donated from eleven different donors. She was lucky in having a large, devoted family willing to donate. The cells were being given from many donors with the hope that a "cross-acceptance" might be achieved, allowing one of these donors to offer a future kidney should the donated child-sized one fail. And just prior to the child-sized kidney being transplanted, she received bone marrow cells from the child, with the parents' approval. The child's sacrificed kidney had become, for Gladys, a borrowed bridge to life.

Even though the abdominal cavity is the preferred place for a kidney transplant, Joe and Franny decided that Gladys had received such severe radiation doses that it would be wiser to put the graft in her thigh, where it could be surgically placed easily and readily observed.

The transplant did not work right away. After two weeks, though, Joe and Franny were guardedly elated as the kidney began to excrete urine. Gladys's family realized that a transplant was their last hope, and when it seemed it might indeed be successful, everyone experienced a moment of relief. By then the nurses and other doctors had melded into a family.

Everyone was rooting for Gladys. But twenty-eight days after the transplant, things began to change. Her white blood cell count fell. The infused marrow did not function. Abnormal bleeding began. She was protected from the threat of infection by living in the sterile environment of the operating room, so no infection to the kidney was evident, but efforts to increase her blood clotting failed. "The balance of survival had tipped over the wrong way," Franny noted.

This was the most practical kidney transplant procedure known at the time, and it had not worked. Despite Gladys's courage, she died. As Franny described, "She died of bleeding because the coagulating power of her blood was lost—an ironic complication of the radiation administered in a vain effort to save her life." At her death, her kidney was still working and was free of rejection.

No method of suppressing antibody production had yet offered a prospect of success for transplanting organs or tissues between those who were not identical twins.

Gladys died as any survivor of nuclear war would eventually die: radiation sickness. Her immune system, deactivated, had been rendered too weak to sustain life.

Joe grieved with her family. Franny took comfort in the lessons that could lead to a method to extend transplantation. He hoped to expand this new shift in treatment to any person doomed to death by the failure of a kidney. And he also found comfort in Emerson's essay "Compensation," in which the great thinker wrote: "Every excess causes a defect; every defect an excess . . . with every influx of light comes new danger. . . . There is a crack in everything God has made."

But Joe was hit hard by the loss of Gladys. "We came so close," he said.

So close.

23

"Some Have Wondered Why We Continued . . ."

CARING FOR GLADYS HAD DRAINED JOE. He had ridden the ups and downs of her daily adjustment in their attempts to give her a borrowed life, and then all hope had disappeared. All the while, he was squeezing in private patients, serving on committees, spending long hours in his lab. He had always been skinny. Soon, he was rail thin. The playful look in his eye became muted and lost light.

It was not that his optimism abandoned him, it was just that his soul was bruised. His energy was frayed. Even his former colleague who'd hired him as a partner straight out of training, Dr. Cannon, noticed. Everyone agreed, Joe did not look well.

Franny was worried. He consulted with Bobby. They both knew that Joe needed a rest. Together, they confronted Joe, telling him to take time off. Take a month. Go away. Start a new habit of a month off every year. No human, even of Joe's extraordinary grit and compassion, could maintain a year round assault against death. His well of strength required refilling on a mandated schedule. No normal human could continue at such an intense pace, not even Joe.

Too tired to put up a fight, he accepted their guidance. Two days after Franny and Bobby talked to him, he drove with Bobby to Woods Hole on Cape Cod and got on the first ferry that came along.

He thought it would be an adventure to get off at one of the islands and explore.

As soon as he set foot on Martha's Vineyard, he was captured by its charm. In a matter of hours, he and Bobby were talking to a realtor about rentals. Learning that those who lived in Edgartown often ferried over to Chappaquiddick Island to swim, Joe decided he wanted to do the exact opposite: rent a house in Chappaquiddick and ferry back to Edgartown for supplies.

During the month in their rented house with Bobby and their children, playing tennis every day, flying kites, picnicking, and swimming, Joe was beginning to feel more like his old self. He also knew that the island would be a part of the rest of his life. Somehow, some time, he would find land there to call his, to live on. It would be his place of restoration, the place where he could feel nature working its miracles, sharing its cycles with the reminders that he was part of the cosmic seasons, too.

His love of humor returned. His love of seeing the comic in the ordinary, his innate playfulness, was like a vine twining with his optimism to soothe the heartrending moments when he could not preserve life for one of his patients. Now the sources of joy he found in his youth to sustain his strength became the storehouse he drew from. In college, he loved to memorize poetry. Each day on the island, lines from the poems he had committed to memory in those years visited his mind, reminding him of a source of comfort that soon he began adding to, word by word, from new poems. Soon he was regaling his family at dinner with recitations of his favorites, including the story of Sam McGee, the fictional Alaskan gold-rusher who died of the cold, but woke with a smile as he was being cremated . . . he was finally warm!

At times he would recall those patients whose courage had left an indelible mark, in particular Charles Woods. His memories of treating Charles at Valley Forge always prompted him to ask if he himself would have the dignity and confidence to walk out into the world with a disfigurement that caused people to stare at him for the rest of his life. And he honestly answered, "I don't know." He knew only that Charles had taught him what a human being can achieve in dealing with adversity. And now he himself was challenged to restore an energy damaged by overwork and sorrow.

He recalled his lifelong fascination with Wilder's play *Our Town*. As he sat at the dining room table, he looked at the faces of his and Bobby's five children—the sixth yet to arrive—savoring the moment, stamping it in his memory.

Soon he was feeling ready to return to work. He held the knowledge of how to keep himself protected and felt ready to move forward, to tackle once again the problem of the human body staving off death by accepting a borrowed organ. He took heart in remembering Louis Pasteur's belief that "science and the application of science are linked together as a fruit to the tree that has borne it."

He walked into the Brigham. His step had a childlike skip.

By now the Brigham was known worldwide as the innovative center for end-stage renal disease. The most desperate patients sought treatment there. As soon as Joe returned to his office, he found another drastic case waiting for him. A twelve-year-old Swedish boy had fallen from a wooden horse on a merry-go-round, rupturing his kidney. Like Gladys, he was found to have been born with only one. Flown quickly to the Brigham, he was given dialysis, which brought him close to everyday well-being. He was moving around, eating, and feeling well. Yet everyone knew there was no long-term hope for him. He could not live without a transplant.

This time, a new factor could be counted on: his donor would be his mother.

Tests showed that the genetic relationship was close. Furthermore, the mother was ready to provide bone marrow cells. After many had been withdrawn from her pelvic bones, she agreed to have a rib removed to provide more cells. The rib was stripped of its marrow cells, which were injected into her son's bloodstream.

The boy was then wheeled into the X-ray room, where he received heavy irradiation and injection of more of his mother's bone marrow cells. The prospect for the transplant seemed exceptionally good. The mother's kidney would be close in genetic compatibility; her marrow cells would adjust his immune system to thinking it was like hers. The gift of her kidney should thrive once it was transplanted. All systems seemed to signal *go*.

Despite great hope from the transplant team, the boy's condition worsened. The bone marrow did not take. His blood count fell to perilously low levels. He was failing so quickly that Joe and the team decided it was not wise to remove the mother's kidney to give to him. There was no reason to endanger her well-being. After twenty-five days of trying to prepare the boy for a transplant, he died.

The loss was hard. Everyone had tried so diligently. Joe and Franny and the transplant team now believed that "even with very dangerous levels of irradiation and an ideal marrow donation, the method was rarely if ever going to be practical: the balance of survival was just too difficult to achieve."

All those in the irradiation experimental trial died. The loss of life was battering to the nurses and interns who spent so much time with those fighting for their lives. One medical resident resigned from the service, saying he could not involve himself any longer. He even went so far as to say he had officiated at enough murders.

Franny and Joe, with nephrologist John Merrill, urological surgeon John Hartwell Harrison, and the chief of medicine, George Thorn, were determined to push on. Taking heart in their belief that the situation would change, they learned from each failure. So close, so close, each time, so close. They knew they had to keep on. Indeed, despite the deaths, a new pattern of the transplanted kidney emerged: each time, the organ functioned longer than expected. It showed few signs of rejection. Death came not from a rejected kidney but from the complications of it: uncontrollable bleeding or the whole-body infection, sepsis.

The frightening powers of irradiation were clear. Heavily inactivating the immune system opened a door to complications that imperiled survival.

They had to find a better way. But they were so close.

Joe wrote, "Some have wondered why we continued in the face of so many failed attempts. I was never discouraged. If we gave up, patients would have no hope at all."

By then, the success of eighteen identical twin transplants was leading the way. These successes were Joe's beacon. He knew there was a better way to affect the immune system, to trick it to receive a foreign tissue as "self," than total body X-ray and bone marrow infusion. He felt certain they would one day create an environment in which a borrowed kidney could thrive. He and his colleagues just had to find it.

24

"Thanks for the Second Drink"

EVERY DAY, THE TEAM AT THE BRIGHAM heard pleas for help from patients dying of renal failure. The dialysis program resorted to receiving only those with a promising outcome. The need outpaced the machines and manpower.

The heartrending decision of whom to accept and whom to turn away fell on Joe and Franny and others on the transplant team. And other issues arose. Like anything anywhere in human endeavor, the prospect of making money from a human need led to the formation of a company with stockholders. This perceived exploitation of the helpless brought outcries from community activists. The Brigham and Harvard Medical School soon disengaged their interests, and John Merrill resigned as a consultant to the company. He preferred remaining on the medical school faculty with its scientific interests rather than work in the business world with its for-profit goals.

This difference in values would eventually lead to the twenty-first-century blurring of lines between hospital chains and medical practices, with the danger that attention is paid as much to making money as to treating disease. And while the early Brigham patients did not face that situation, the need for the Brigham to cover the costs of its innovative, risky program had its own challenge. The early patients gave a substantial amount to be considered for a transplant. In the trials to seek methods to control rejection, the National Institutes of Health helped. Also, the Heart Fund gave, since heart failure was a complication of renal disease. Brigham patients and their families formed the Kidney Transplant/Dialysis Association. They raised money through bake sales, raffles, and any other fundraisers they could think up. In time, they provided a patients' lounge and bought the hospital more equipment. And, of course, the desire to find treatments for survivors of nuclear war helped fund the irradiation trials.

———————

JANUARY 1959, a month much waited for. An unexpected success came; the dark years were relieved. The grim past, when Joe and Franny and the transplant team watched their patients die of radiation sickness, succumbing to bleeding and infection, was now to be brightened. And it started with John Riteris.

He came from Wisconsin. He traveled to the Brigham suffering from glomerulonephritis and the double hit of a bacterial infection. Like so many others, he came hoping for hope. The intriguing part of what Riteris offered Joe and the transplant team was that John had a twin. Not an identical one, but a twin, nonetheless. Furthermore, Andrew, the healthy twin, came with his dying brother to the Brigham, already decided. He had no anxiety about it. He was ready and willing to give one of his healthy kidneys to his brother and considered it a done deal.

Joe and Franny took one glance at the pair and instantly knew they were not identical. They were of different heights. They had different hair color. Their body structures were different. Their birth records showed that they were born seven minutes apart, and each had weighed six and a half pounds. The physician who delivered them noted that there had been two placentas, one for each twin, which made it certain that they were dizygotic: twins from two separate eggs rather than from one that had split. They would not have the likelihood of success the Herrick identical twins enjoyed.

From what Peter had learned from bovine cattle, and from his studies that put the workings of the immune system on display, it was now clear how immunity worked with pre-birth sharing of tissues through one placenta. No one yet knew how John's body would respond when it was faced with a kidney graft from his brother Andrew. The prospects of their tissues bypassing rejection were a roll of the dice.

As predictable and logical as science may be, there is always a gap through which the unexpected slips in, only to be explained later. So it had been with Charles's long-lasting skin grafts, which Joe viewed as a scientific phenomenon. By now, Joe accepted his assumption that Charles's immune system had been too depleted to attack the foreign skin from a cadaver in the usual time. But what would happen when Andrew's kidney was transplanted into John, he could not predict.

For that reason alone, the case was enthralling: a clear chance for Franny and Joe to learn more about the acceptance of borrowed tissue. The fact that they also had the chance to save John's life was the most compelling. Toward that end, they came up with a treatment plan revised from their former failures. They would give light doses of irradiation, skip the marrow transplant, and go from there.

They admitted the Riteris brothers for a potential transplant.

After stabilizing John with dialysis, Joe performed a skin graft between them. The graft on Andrew's arm showed immunological rejection after twelve days, proof that they were not identical twins. A second was applied. The identity of the twins was now clearly established, especially when Andrew's second graft was more quickly rejected than the first, as predicted by Peter's discovery of the second set phenomenon. There was definite genetic closeness, though not the assured compatibility of the Herrick twins' transplant.

Even though the blood group between them was similar, it was not identical. With these findings, Joe and Franny and the transplant team began preparing John for Andrew's kidney.

Twice John lay under the X-ray machine to receive whole-body irradiation. Then the surgery was scheduled. When one of Andrew's healthy kidneys was removed, Joe placed it in John's abdomen. He used the exact techniques he had perfected for the Herrick twins' surgery. Right away, the borrowed kidney dripped urine. Again, the transplant team celebrated, yet with restraint since so many other times a transplanted kidney had eventually stopped working. The prospect of the patient's survival threatened everyone on the team; loss would never be accepted as normal.

This time, and for the first time, the one dying of renal disease did not falter from the irradiation. John's white blood cell count fell, but he did not develop the dreaded radiation sickness.

The transplanted kidney began working like a steam engine. In fact, it began producing too much liquid waste, and though it felt like a triumph, it was actually a sign that John's kidney was a bit sick. A normal kidney controls the amount of fluid filtered through it each day, and the borrowed kidney was not regulating itself as it should. To keep John from becoming dangerously dehydrated, Joe and Franny made sure that he received intravenous sterile saline.

Thankfully, over the next few days, John's new kidney got a grip on the fluid it was filtering, and the transplant team began to guardedly celebrate again. Yet, no sooner had another day passed than things changed. John spiked a fever. Now critically ill from the infection in his own two kidneys, which were still in place, he was rushed to middle-of-the-night surgery.

Just nineteen days after whole-body irradiation and eleven days after the transplant, Dr. Harrison removed both of John's heavily infected kidneys. John was again fighting for his life. Franny said, "It was one of the most critical operations in the entire kidney transplant experience."

The response was remarkable. John was soon feeling well, eating everything in sight, and maintaining a normal temperature—a sign there was no infection.

Then, nine months after the transplant, the smoldering process of rejection began. Quickly, Joe and the team put John on cortisone and gave him a small dose of whole-body irradiation. They continued this treatment weekly for four more weeks. And a remarkable thing happened—all signs of rejection retreated.

Soon, John was feeling well again; normal, in fact. Now began the real celebration, *and* the mystery. What had allowed this to happen? For years, Joe and the team had hoped for exactly this outcome, but it was always thought that rejection could not be reversed. It was assumed that once the body turned on the foreign tissue of a transplanted kidney, there would be no way to make the body change course.

Unless foreign tissue was borrowed from an identical twin, it was impossible for the body to stop turning against the borrowed organ and begin to accept it as "self." But here was proof that the scientific assumption had been wrong. Rejection had been reversed.

This was a pivotal moment in transplantation history. The barrier had been broken. John Riteris was the first human being in whom the immune system's exquisite power had been manipulated. Joe and the team's publication in the *Journal of the American Medical Association* in 1963 declared that the success of this transplant between nonidentical brothers broke "the genetic barriers . . . and became in principle the single most important case, psychologically and otherwise, in the history of the field of clinical transplantation. Within weeks, a group in Paris confirmed the Brigham's findings by successfully placing kidneys from fraternal twins into their radiated siblings. One died, but the other would live for 26 years."

Franny and Joe believed they had made a monumental step forward. But the outcome soon became suspect. Other transplant programs pointed out that the whole-body irradiation given to John had been slight, that the dose had not been large enough to depress the immune system for long. Such a mild course of irradiation shouldn't have achieved John's remarkable ability to accept his brother's kidney.

Worldwide discussion followed. The case of John Riteris was finally accepted as a random success. Franny said it was "like hitting the jackpot in a slot machine." He suspected that while the twins were developing in the womb, they must have at some point shared a common blood supply despite the evidence that they had two placentas. The miracle of birth always holds onto its secrets.

As for Joe, he simply accepted that not all answers could be known. He later remarked, "As a doctor, I now know that it is not necessary to know everything. If a patient—even just a single patient—survives with good quality of life that means a lot. As a scientist, I may have been unhappy with the human X-ray protocol, but as the physician in charge of John's care, I was ecstatic . . . delighted that things had gone so well."

So well, in fact, that John would live another twenty-nine years.

John himself, as one who had felt his life fading and believed he was doomed, only to wake one day to the sudden rush of his life force returning, lived in awe of his good fortune and what had been done for him. Andrew downplayed his part, saying he always believed the contribution of a donor is not an unusual one—"that it is nothing more than the rare chance to be a Good Samaritan to one's kin."

As strange as it may seem, he and John never really talked about it. They always found ways to talk around it, as brothers are apt to do.

But then, two decades later, John wrote a letter. "To Andrew—thanks for the second drink."

25

Send in the Dogs

JOE REALIZED THAT he and the transplant team had been going down a side road. The X-ray/bone marrow method was too dangerous. They needed a better protocol to prepare someone dying of renal failure for a borrowed kidney. However, important things had been learned. Improving one patient's care added to the care of another. Also, to reach the holy grail of transplanting an organ from an unrelated cadaver, it was clear that a new, safer way had to be found.

In 1959, Joe read in *Nature* the work of Dr. Robert Schwartz and Dr. William Dameshek, hematologists at Tufts Medical School in Boston, about the effects on the immune system of an anticancer drug called 6-MP. It was synthesized by biochemists George Hitchings and Gertrude Elion at a private company in New York as they engaged in a lifelong study of the building blocks of proteins.

Their studies had been simple. Rabbits were given 6-MP along with a foreign protein that normally caused antibodies to be produced against it. When both the drug and foreign protein were given together, the rabbits failed to make antibodies against the invading proteins while retaining the ability to make antibodies against other invading proteins. Bingo! The rabbits did not become "immunological cripples."

This drug would be ideal for combating the deadly effects of lowering the power of the immune system by irradiation. Knock out one invader, but keep the power to knock out others. Perfect: 6-MP fooled the immune system with no deadly side effects.

This was a striking finding.

Joe declared himself "a willing convert." He believed the drugs were the way to go, but John Merrill did not wholeheartedly agree. While Joe had constant "hands-on" connection with his lab— where methods were tried and either discarded or kept—John did not have the personal experience of witnessing Joe's results. John had spent a year in Paris working closely with a transplant team whose belief in X-irradiation had strongly influenced him.

Peter, however, believed in a drug protocol and sent a research fellow from his lab to Joe's. On his way to Boston, the fellow visited Hitchings and Elion in Tuckahoe, New York, where they had synthesized 6-MP as well as other drugs for Joe to use in studies.

Joe also traveled to Tuckahoe to learn firsthand from the chemists who were making these groundbreaking discoveries. The dogs in Joe's lab became not just transplant warriors but heroes, the bearers of innovated breakthroughs. Sam, a beagle mix, took on irradiation and bone marrow infusion from a donor in hopes of preparing a receptive immune system for a transplant. And he, like Gladys Loman, succumbed to losing his balance of protection. After forty-nine days, he died of distemper.

With the discovery of drugs that could convince the immune system to become gracious hosts to transplanted foreign tissue, the laboratory dogs became famous pioneers. Honest John, another beagle mix, was prepared for a transplant by whole-body irradiation and marrow cells from his donor, then maintained on the immuno-suppressive drug methotrexate. In the next few years, Honest John would still be bounding around the research laboratory with his transplanted kidney.

A larger beagle mix named New Hampshire facilitated a remarkable breakthrough in the Harvard Medical School Surgical Research Lab when he was given a kidney transplant and maintained on the drug azathioprine. He not only kept his kidney, he was scurrying around the laboratory becoming well known to all experimenters in the transplant field. He did so well that Joe and his lab staff tied a ribbon around his neck and had a party. But his contribution was not yet over. Two years after his transplant, he was photographed and shown on television. The friendly yellow and white mutt inspired the transplant field worldwide—and gave it great hope—as his immunosuppressive drug had been stopped and he continued to thrive. New Hampshire enabled the belief that one day, as the immunosuppressive drugs became more sophisticated, it would be possible to suspend the use of the drug in human patients as well.

Mona, a medium-sized brown-and-white beagle mix, offered supreme proof that drugs would be the way of the future. When she was given a borrowed kidney and placed on the drug azathioprine, she thrived and delivered a large litter of healthy puppies.

Joe knew that without these studies on animals, a successful human organ transplant never would have happened. They became pets of the laboratory workers, always fed and exercised, and cared for in the best ways possible. There was an open door policy for visitors to the labs, especially veterinary students who learned a great deal about surgical procedures.

By the early sixties, dogs on the drug Imuran were successfully carrying their transplanted kidneys and frolicking in the outdoor courtyards. It was time, Joe thought, to adapt the Imuran protocols to humans. The X-ray strategy followed by bone-marrow transfusion was now considered a side road. Research in drug-induced immunological tolerance had replaced it.

Donald Toby was only twenty-two, dying of renal failure, when he appeared at the Brigham. And he was big, so big that no one knew how much of the immunosuppressive drugs to give him. No past experience could give guidance. Extrapolating the amounts from dog to man was complicated.

After Donald's transplant in March 1961, the same dosage of Imuran that was given to transplanted dogs was administered to Donald. He was the first patient to be treated with the new drug. For the first few weeks after the surgery, Joe thought they'd hit a home run. Donald's new kidney, donated through Don Matson's sacrificed-kidney surgery, began pouring out gallons of urine. The transplant team watched with glee.

Four weeks later, Donald was still thriving. But on the twenty-ninth day, infection started. Joe realized the immunosuppressive dose had been too high. Tragically, Donald's bone marrow function was destroyed. He died, not from organ rejection, but from drug toxicity. As with Gladys Loman, the loss was brutal.

The team was deeply saddened. And dejected.

After two more deaths, even with the drug dosage halved, despite the blow of failure and loss, Joe intuitively felt they were within close reach of success. They couldn't stop. Lessons learned from the loss of these courageous pioneer-patients guided them. They kept banging on the door of scientific exploration, following one theory, discarding it, taking up another, refining it, placing it under the scrutiny of statistics and a reasonable longing to restore life. Life, not just for one, but for untold thousands. *That* seemed only inches from their grasp.

Then, the moment.

26

"It Was a Good Time to Be Alive"

IN EARLY JANUARY 1962, a twenty-three-year-old man was desperate. In and out of the Brigham for dialysis, he was dying of renal failure from glomerulonephritis. Working as an accountant, he was trying to keep up his schedule. Dialysis helped, but it could not maintain his life for long.

From the days when Kolff fashioned a means to wash blood with tomato cans and sausage casing to the construction of barrel-sized machines that sat beside a patient, the dialysis work of engineers and medical scientists had worked its magic. So for Mel Doucette, Joe's patient, dialysis treatment was able to be administered through a button-sized hole in the wall of his abdomen, through which the blood's waste products could be removed.

It was a clever design, replacing the dialysis machine's membrane with the use of the body's own peritoneum—the thin membrane that covers the intestines—to wash toxins from the blood. This way, a patient could feel well for longer periods, have daily painless treatments, and stay at home to live a somewhat normal life. At least for a while.

The danger was infection. Also, over time, the treatment became less and less effective. Sooner or later, patients realized that only a transplant could save them. And such was the case for Mel.

He had no twin. He had no family members eligible to be a donor. He lived in the Brigham on dialysis, desperate for a kidney to become available.

For a week, Joe slept in the hospital. Two other doctors also stayed overnight on the transplant unit, hoping that through a death from injury a compatible kidney for Mel would be found. Three times, it seemed an organ was available; but each time, the match fell through. Then on April 5, the chance came.

With heartbreak for the family but elation for Mel and determination for Joe, a message came from the operating room. A thirty-year-old man had just died while his heart was being repaired. At the close of the operation, his heart would not resume its normal beat, and, at the moment of death, both of his kidneys were functioning well.

Since his body was being cooled in a state of hypothermia to minimize the risks to his diseased heart, both of his kidneys were in a state of suspension. Their blood supply was merely waiting to be resumed. It was fortunate coincidence that the deceased man's red blood cell type was compatible with Mel's. With other crucial tests, such as finding no infection in the kidney, and no history of kidney disease, the transplant team sprang into action.

Joe met with the grieving family. Despite their sadness, they permitted the transplant team to take one of the young man's kidneys for Mel. With time being so critical, the operating room cleared its schedule for that night. The cadaver kidney was removed, cooled further, and after forty minutes, Joe was placing it into Mel, using the same surgical techniques he had perfected for the transplant between the Herrick twins. This time, however, the borrowed organ had no relation to Mel.

All of the staff were aware of this historical moment. The ultimate goal of transplantation that Joe had been hoping to reach for nearly a decade was here.

When the surgery was completed, Mel was immediately placed on an immunosuppressive drug. Franny noted that the cooling of the transplanted organ was clearly in the borrowed kidney's favor, as it had been without circulation for two full hours, which ordinarily would have been damaging. Now the crucial time came. Joe and the team were in uncharted territory. The decisions Joe wrestled with brought real anguish. He knew the treatment that followed could cost Mel his life.

It was also essential that Joe and John Merrill work together to settle on the best course. Their decisions could mean the difference in Mel's chances to hold onto his borrowed kidney or in tipping him over into losing it—and with it, his life. To Joe, the intellectual rivalry between them was like a tennis match, as they volleyed opinions back and forth.

Murray: Treat him only with Imuran.

Merrill: Increase his dosage.

Murray: But we don't want to lose him to drug toxicity.

Merrill: Give small doses of whole-body irradiation in place of actinomycin.

Murray: That seems too hazardous. I argue for the continuation of our present course   actinomycin weekly, Imuran daily.

Which is what they did.

Despite their debates, the teamwork was extraordinary. All the staff were aware of the historic value of this case. Outside Mel's room, they would disagree, discussing his treatment. But then they would unite in warm, personal support of his well-being.

On the fifth day after surgery, Mel's borrowed kidney began working. Things looked bright. *Hope* took wing. For the next three weeks, chances looked good. The borrowed kidney worked like an engine, gaining speed. The transplant team guardedly celebrated, knowing that, as in previous times—indeed, in all human ground-breaking endeavors—trouble was likely slinking around at the edges, ready to break in. Yet optimism spread. There were days worthy of celebrating. Minute by minute was the measure.

Suddenly, dark energy pushed through, snipping at Mel's chances. On the thirty-ninth day, he spiked a high fever and became severely ill. He had all the signs that his body was rejecting his new kidney.

But by now Joe and Franny knew they were not powerless at an immobile rejection barrier. They could move the barrier. They had learned they could turn rejection from its course. They just had to find the right solution. Continuing to give the drug Imuran, they now adjusted the amount of actinomycin.

The crisis subsided. Soon it became clear that Mel's diseased kidneys weren't doing him any good. The team decided to remove them. Taking out diseased kidneys was always a hard decision. If the borrowed kidney completely failed, Mel would be totally bare of the essential organs to maintain life. There was always the chance that his diseased kidneys could tide him over with dialysis until another borrowed kidney would be found. But now it seemed best to get the old kidneys out of the way.

In two surgeries Dr. Harrison removed them. No sooner were they gone than another immunologic rejection crisis erupted.

The drugs Mel had been given did not seem to be holding the transplanted kidney in a safe environment. A third was added: cortisone. As a hormone naturally produced in the body, cortisone affects the ability of an antibody to attack an antigen. In Cushing syndrome, identified and named by Harvey Cushing, too much is produced. In its synthetic chemical form, cortisone was found to be able to reverse rejection in a transplant patient. Which with Mel, it did.

Soon again, trouble rattled the gates, forcing its way in. Mel developed pneumonia. The dark energy kept nipping.

The saving guide turned out to be dog studies. Kennel diseases had been overcome in transplanted canines by using antibiotics. In spite of the dogs being on an immunosuppressive drug, they had been successfully treated for an assortment of infections from kennel cough to pneumonia. Following that history, antibiotics were now given to Mel.

Again, he was saved. His blood pressure returned to normal. His borrowed kidney was still working, keeping him well. Though it did not function as a healthy one, he was at least feeling well enough to enjoy a nearly normal life and went back to work.

The dark head of trouble would not be still, though. It burst through again. This time, Mel had appendicitis!

Of course the badly infected appendix had to be removed. Even after it was out, Mel's condition remained stormy. Day by day, he improved. Little by little, he rallied. He got up and went home.

He seemed as well as ever. He was still on the drugs that kept rejection in check, and for months he lived in comfort. But toward the end of January, the signs of the worst thing that could happen began to be seen: the borrowed kidney was failing.

On January 22, twenty-one months after his transplant, Joe gave Mel a second kidney. This time the borrowed organ came from one of Don's patients, a child whose surgery required the sacrifice of a kidney.

It took. It worked. It thrived. As knowledge of Mel's restoration to good health spread throughout kidney transplant centers, the number of patients operated on increased. Transplantation was now accepted as a lifesaving measure.

Joe published Mel's case in the *New England Journal of Medicine* in June 1963. This was a milestone that had long been hoped for. It was now that the medical profession began to think of transplanting an organ *not* as a wild prospect to save a dying patient but as an acceptable treatment for end-stage renal disease. Borrowing organs was no longer seen as science fiction or a foolish idea hatched from Americans' love for ingenuity and innovation.

Surgeons and scientists reveled in America's reputation for having an abundance of creativity and pioneering courage.

On the one-year mark of Mel's operation, when he was still well, still taking immunosuppressive drugs to keep his body hospitable to his borrowed kidney, Joe felt like tying a ribbon around his neck. Instead, he savored the timeline. In just eight years from when the Herrick twins walked into the Brigham doors in 1954, and eighteen years from the day Charles's long-lasting skin grafts aroused his curiosity, he had reached the "holy grail": a successful transplantation of an organ from a deceased donor to an unrelated doomed patient. The triumph was like a flood of light.

The success washed over Joe's memories of days when those hanging on to hope by sheer grit and the thread of a prayer had bravely put their trust in him. Ultimately, they had given their lives to him, not on the battlefield in the war that set Joe on this path, but in the conquest to preserve life—which, in its most essential form, is the simple turning of hours, the shedding of days. To that end, Joe's dedication was now preserving life for thousands.

RECOGNITION CAME to the transplant team, at least for Franny. On May 8, 1963, *Time Magazine* came out with a banner across the top right corner saying, *If they can operate, you're lucky.* Franny's portrait filled the cover.

He wore a surgical cap, scrubs, and an untied mask that dangled around his neck. His eyes looked down in intense concern and concentration. Floating in the air around him were surgical instruments—scissors, files, retractors—all things that looked like torture instruments except that they were the magical means to man-made miracles. Franny was now forty-nine, at the pinnacle of his career.

In the sixteen-page spread, the magazine described seven major operations transforming medicine, highlighting the pioneering surgeons Lillehei and Debakey for heart surgery; Cooper for brain surgery for tremors in Parkinson's disease; Urban for using lymph nodes in a new approach in breast cancer surgery; Sakellarides for orthopedic surgery for the reconstruction of arthritic hands; Schuknecht for ear surgery through a microscope. And Franny. He was featured as following in the footsteps of the great surgeons Harvey Cushing and William Halstead, who transformed general surgery from an earlier era. Furthermore, the article pointed out that Franny was practicing when "American surgery was poised to leap ahead as Europe's medical centers lost some of their best brains to Hitler's anti-Semitism and to World War II." He was said to be among the new surgeons moving away from the "era of the great man in surgery, dominated by the European system when the great man seldom saw the patient before an operation."

A brief history was woven in, describing how early surgeons wore a gown with striped pants and "operated swiftly with never an unnecessary stroke of the scalpel or a needless word to his assistants and nurses. When he had cut out what had to be cut out, he departed and left an assistant to close the surgical wound, which was the usual protocol until the 1930s."

The article featured Franny as one of those breaking that tradition, one who watched over his patient from preparation through postoperative care, "taking care of the whole patient."

Of course, the Herrick twins' kidney transplant was among the innovative operations featured, along with the search to suppress the immune reaction to a kidney transplanted from a cadaver. The article even went on to add, "The moment a method is found to control the immune mechanism in man, there will be a flood of transplants of many organs." And an illustration humorously used a picture of the Tin Man in *The Wizard of Oz* sporting the sentence, "Spare parts may be available."

In describing the groundbreaking Herrick transplant, much was made of the roles played by Merrill, Harrison, and Thorn, with little mention of Joe. The article even mistakenly cited Dr. David Hume as placing Ronald's donated kidney into Richard. Franny was distraught over the error since he was the one who had been in contact with the *Time* editor. And he apologized to Joe.

Joe absorbed the slight but hoped it would be corrected. Secretly, he feared slipping out of transplant history. Despite his gentle, understated temperament, he had the usual amount of ambition. He did not want to be forgotten. He did not want to vanish from transplant history.

As soon as the magazine was on the newsstands, Franny's phone began to ring. He marveled at his colleagues' reactions—some proud that their profession was receiving favorable attention; others showing envy; others hurt that they were left out, "feeling more worthy of such prominent mention." Some accused him of seeking the attention. He summed it up as "reactions [ranging] from sweet grapes to sour grapes and then to grapes of wrath." But he was pleased that the majority of his colleagues gave him the sort of backing one needs "when you are suddenly thrust into a spotlight position of unwonted and unwanted prominence."

To Americans in 1963, transplanting organs was titillating. The average man and woman thought of it as shocking, weird, disorienting, and rather comforting. If some body part hit the skids, there was now the prospect that a spare could be found. That was how most thought of it. The work that had consumed much of Joe, Franny, and Peter's lives had remained offstage, separated from the daily knowledge of ordinary life. For those suffering from renal disease, it had always been different. For many, transplantation had been their only hope to stay alive. And now for many others, it was their only glimpse of a future. In the three decades between that article and Joe's winning of the Nobel Prize, some 200,000 human kidney transplants would be successfully performed. And the success with kidney transplants would transfer to the borrowing of heart, lung, liver, and skin—new organs that did more than staving off death: they preserved life.

In November of that year, after the *Time* cover story had blown over, Franny was duck-hunting with friends in Maine when the wife of their farmer hunting guide rushed a half mile from the house, shouting, "The president's been shot!" Although Franny was four years younger, and in a later class at Harvard, he had known President Kennedy. In the middle of the 1940s, when the Boston Chamber of Commerce selected several young men who were "coming up fast," he and Kennedy met at a dinner held in their honor. JFK was a congressman at that time. With the assassination, Franny was jolted, feeling a personal loss. He drove back home listening to the radio all the way, grieving that one of his own generation had been killed "in the line of duty."

The tragedy, he felt, thrust the era into uncertainty, and he decided the best remedy for his grief was work. The *Time* article had heralded the new age of transplantation, and he was still firmly anchored in the field, now focusing his knowledge on pioneering a liver transplant. What the article could not convey were the years and years of failures, attempts, more failures, and the inch-by-inch movement forward, which often felt like scrambling in the dark for the day the rejection barrier would be broken.

There was no way for readers to know what it had felt like for Joe and Franny, as well as others on the team, to watch over their brave and dying patients, who were holding onto hope, what Emily Dickinson called "the thing with feathers that perches in the soul."

There was also no way for the general reader to know what those years were like for ones dying of renal failure, wishing for some magical charm to help them hang onto the kidneys that had been transplanted in a Hail Mary attempt to save their lives. The magic charm materialized for them in the sight of Joe, Franny, and the others coming to care for them.

From the day that Joe witnessed Charles's skin grafts lasting longer than expected, inspiring the question *Why not transplant organs to save a life as well?*, the rejection battle had been the front line in the war to borrow life. Franny, Joe, and Peter had been those leaders to dig in, to never look up, to never falter or retreat.

Three decades later, after Franny nominated Joe for the Nobel Prize in Medicine, Joe would say in his acceptance speech, "My only wish would be to have ten more lives to live on this planet. I'd spend one in embryology, genetics, physics, astronomy, and geology. The other as a pianist, backwoodsman, tennis player, or writer for the *National Geographic*. And I'd keep one open for another life-time as a surgeon-scientist."

Franny viewed their quest humbly. He saw it as one of compassion, but also one of wonder. He liked to recall the feeling he had when he performed his very first surgery as a young surgeon just out of training, doing a simple (but then, they are never completely simple) appendectomy on a twelve-year-old boy, a boy whose well-being had been snapped in two in moments. "Here I was, with skilled nurses and shiny sterile instruments at hand, ready to operate. I felt that this was both a miracle and a privilege."

As humbly, they walked away from winning their war, leaving a lasting mark in the annals of history, we might imagine them tipping their hats and giving their last words to Peter, who said succinctly in his favorite style—*It was a good time to be alive.*

Epilogue

THE LAST NORMAL day that Peter and Jean Medawar spent together was Saturday, September 6, 1969. They were in Exeter in the southwest of England for the British Association, an esteemed group founded in 1831 for the advancement of science and the enrichment of its lay members. As president of the association, Peter was scheduled to give a speech on Saturday and read a lesson at a service at Exeter Cathedral on Sunday. He had worked for months on his speech, as well as on the organization's program of lectures. All week he'd been talking to reporters, surrounded by people wanting either his opinion or help.

On Friday, he delivered his address using Sir Francis Bacon's essay, "On the Effecting of All Things Possible," as a point of departure. As he neared the end, his connection with his audience was palpable. His voice swelled to his conclusion, in which he cited Thomas Hobbes's likening life to a race with no finishing post. "The great thing is to be in it, to be a contestant in the attempt to make the world a better place . . . to forsake the course is to die." After his last word, a hush fell over the lecture hall, then a roaring applause swelled and seemed as if it would never stop.

Jean wasn't surprised. Sitting in the audience, she had felt the same reaction at home when Peter tried out the speech on her. Thinking it the "best and most splendid statement on human aspirations that she had ever read or heard," she had burst into tears.

Her emotional response didn't stun Peter, because he himself was extremely moved by words.

Ordinarily, after his presidential address, he would be free to relax. But one of the invited lecturers sent word that he could not attend, so to keep the meeting flowing smoothly, Peter agreed to stand in for him, and he gave the second lecture extemporaneously, drawing on his own wide-ranging knowledge, but also using energy he had not prepared to use.

The next day, Jean convinced him to take a long walk. They hiked to the River Dart, with its pool of water the color of tea. It was so serene and lovely, Jean jumped in. Peter followed, coming out dripping, saying, "That was wonderful. I feel much better. We must come back tomorrow after the service and do it again."

However, his mood didn't last long. Nor would he ever be able to come back.

He slept fitfully. He woke early on Sunday morning, irritable. When Jean teased him that he'd be off the hook as soon as he read the lesson in the cathedral—traditionally a comment from a scientist on a Biblical verse—he answered her sharply, "I'm in no mood for raillery."

After that, Jean kept quiet. His irritability was out of character, but considering the responsibilities he had taken on, it was understandable. She watched him put on his doctor's robes and walk in procession with the other dignitaries into the cathedral. As he walked up the aisle past her, he blew her a kiss. That moment would prove to be the last time she would see him walk without difficulty. At the lectern he read the lesson, chapter seven of the Wisdom of Solomon, with a firm voice that, as expected, carried throughout the cathedral. Then his voice began to change and slur.

To Jean, it did not seem possible that anything had gone wrong with him. But it had. Terribly wrong. A moment later in horror, she realized he was having a stroke. She climbed across the pews to him. A group of men came to hold up his limp body. Someone called for an ambulance.

For years, Jean had been dreading something like this. The way he drove himself did not seem possible for any human. Now the world had stopped for him, and would be forever changed. Ordinary things would never again be easy. Some would even be impossible. He was only fifty-four.

Over the next months, it was clear that he had lost the use of the left side of his body as well as the vision in the left half of each eye. His mind was spared, as if intelligence as dazzling could not be impaired. With Jean's help, he continued to travel and lecture around the world, always saying, when someone asked how he took pleasure in life with such handicaps, "I have a very decided preference for remaining alive." In later years, he resorted to an electric wheelchair, always working hard to keep his mind sharp and intact.

But two more strokes took their toll, and in October 1987, at the age of seventy-two, he died. Jean and their four children planted a tree in his memory at the Medawar Memorial Grove at Alfriston, England. Jean lived on into her nineties, writing a memoir of their life together titled after what he said so often: *A Very Decided Preference*. She died May 3, 2005, in Hampstead, England.

Soon after Ronald Herrick left the Brigham, he went back to his second year at Worcester State Teachers College. Math was his major, and teaching was his goal. On his way to campus, he often stopped at a variety store to buy a newspaper. One day, the girl behind the cash register told him she had a friend, Cynthia, starting at the state college. And Cynthia needed a ride there. Ronald agreed that after she rode the bus from her hometown of Marlborough to the Northborough bus stop, he'd pick her up there and drive her to campus. He also decided he'd charge her three dollars a week for the lift. The money would come in handy. Besides, he liked the simplicity of a business arrangement.

At dawn on the day that Cynthia climbed on the bus in Marlborough to go to her first day of college classes, her nerves jangled. Would she be able to find her classes? Would she be able to find Ronald Herrick at the bus stop? What if she couldn't recognize his car? She'd been told to look for a green Chevy and a twenty-four-year-old man, a veteran of the Korean War. But what if he wasn't waiting for her?

As her bus pulled up in Northborough, she saw a green car parked at the curb. When she opened the door, she saw a casually dressed young man with brown hair neatly combed. She also made a mental note that he was handsome. "Ronald Herrick?" she asked, shyly.

"Yup. Get in. You must be Cynthia."

He was naturally quiet, made conversation only when he had something to say, inherently serious with a no-nonsense style. When he began asking her questions, it seemed like an interrogation. But his tone was warm, his intentions friendly—clearly. To lighten up his serious nature, he began whistling as he drove. Over the weeks that he gave her the three-dollar lifts, he sometimes hummed or sang. Then one day, he told her, "You'll have to take the bus tomorrow. I have to go to Boston to the hospital." And added, "It's just for some kidney tests."

"Is there something wrong?" Cynthia asked, concerned.

"I hope not," he said, "I have just the one."

"What happened to the other one?"

"I gave it to my brother."

Cynthia was stunned: here, for weeks, she had been sitting

beside this humble young man who had recently made medical history but never mentioned it until now.

Soon, rather than meeting her at the bus stop, he was driving to pick her up at her home. One day, a blue car stopped instead of Ron's green one. When she opened the door, she saw the driver was not Ron but looked so much like him it was uncanny. And mesmerizing. Richard was slightly smaller, his hair a little lighter, and when he spoke his voice was so like Ron's it dazed her in a sense of wonder. "Ron won't be going in until later today, so he asked me to drive you," Richard said, smiling his infectious grin.

Fascinated, Cynthia studied this near-perfect match to Ron: the same hands, the same dimpled chin, the same way he sat while driving, the same songs and whistling. Identical twins are spellbinding by the sheer uniqueness of their existence. But it was Ron whom she thought of as single and unique, the one she had come to know and admire.

Five years later, in 1959, she and Ron married. His man-in-charge, serious personality never wavered. Over the years when he drove her to college, he continued to charge her three dollars each week; it became a running joke in their fifty-one-year marriage.

They taught school in the same town; they moved to Maine; they bought a farm where Ronald reveled in his memories growing up on his grandfather's farm, harvesting hay, caring for dairy cows, loving the rural way of life.

In his high school math classes, his students called him Mr. Herrick. They thought of him as someone who could do square roots in his head—as someone who was never absent from school, as someone who could always be counted on to give a quiz every Friday. Not until the day when a student brought in a biology book with the picture of their math teacher as a young man on a page, explaining that he was the first donor of a successful kidney transplant, did anyone think of him differently. Being famous for being in a biology book was something. He became more than a living calculator who could blindside a student, asking, "What percent of eight is twelve?" Then, again, Mr. Herrick's other means to fame became the day that the school intercom blasted the message: "Mr. Herrick will not be in for the rest of the day. His cattle have stampeded and at this very moment he's riding out to head them off before they destroy downtown."

He and Richard never talked about the biological history they made. For eight years, life for Richard was tinted with the ordinary day-in-day-out of working in a clothing store, being the father to two girls, and living happily with Clare. His girls were just small children when his gifted kidney was struck with the same disease that destroyed his own years before. Seeing him so sick, Ronald and Cynthia visited often. In 1962, throughout his decline, his pleasant personality never faltered. He smiled no matter how he felt. One night at Richard's house, Ronald looked over at Richard's small daughter as if seeing her for the first time. "That one looks like you," he said. Richard looked at her, thought about it, then sat back, smiling sadly.

That was the last time Ronald saw Richard looking well.

By February 1963, he was bedridden. On a Thursday afternoon in March, Ron suddenly appeared outside Cynthia's classroom door. It was only two o'clock, so Cynthia knew that something was wrong. Richard died that day: March 14, 1963. He was thirty-one years old. For Ronald, it would always be from then on as if he lived with a phantom limb.

Today, one of Richard's grown daughters is a dialysis nurse. Her son, people say, so resembles Richard that it brings to mind American poet Maxine Kumin's words in her poem "The Retrieval System": "When I'm alone these features come up to link my lost people."

Clare lived into her eighties, saying she simply did not want to find out what was ailing her; it was time to go. Ronald lived to the age of seventy-nine, when he died of heart failure. Cynthia, as of this writing, is a spry eighty, holding onto memories of Ronald, keeping them vivid and alive. She is the keeper, too, of the courageous lives of the two brothers who made history.

Milan Hašek came to a tragic end after the Russian invasion of Prague. The Communist government squeezed his research findings, revising them to meet their dogma, using his science for propaganda. In 1984, he committed suicide.

No one knew how prophetic Donald Matson's comment would be when Joe asked him "if one of these spare kidneys could be made available for Gladys, and Don jokingly replied that he had been involved in one Nobel Prize venture, now perhaps he'd become involved in another." Joe later fervently wished that Don would have lived to see his prophecy come true. A decade after he gave a child-sized kidney to Joe for Gladys, Don began showing symptoms of Creutzfeldt-Jakob disease (also known as mad cow disease), which he had been researching. Tragically, he may have contracted the fatal illness while consulting on a case. He died May 10, 1969, only fifty-six.

Franny was one of the most, if not the most, eminent surgeons in the world. His academic writings underlined his reputation for surgical excellence. And he loved to write. From his days as a medical student, he discovered his joy in a well-constructed sentence when he wrote articles for historical medical journals. He particularly enjoyed doing car-trip research with Laurie on Civil War medicine. He wrote a total of six books, with his textbook *The*

Metabolic Care of the Surgical Patient, published in 1959, becoming a classic.

By 1972, he was tired. In a conversation with the Harvard Medical School dean, he worked up to the subject of his retirement by starting, "Bob, in July 1973, I will have been head of my department for twenty-five years. And I have always said that no major department of a university should be under the thumb of the same person for more than a quarter of a century." He added, "I think it's time we got a younger man to run the department."

The dean was caught off guard. Then he asked, "When is your Harvard retirement age?"

"June 30, 1981," Franny shot back. Since his faculty appointment had been in 1948, his retirement had been officially set for June 30 after his sixty-seventh birthday.

The dean then bluntly said, "You can't retire now."

"Why?" Franny prompted.

"Because I'm going to retire."

That settled the question. So for four more years, until 1977, Franny kept on as the chief of surgery at the Brigham.

His retirement was not really a retirement; it was merely a branching out of his interests. He spent hours writing and raising funds for building a new hospital merging the Brigham with the Women's Hospital. He was given an office on the fourth floor of the Countway Library. Soon, he was taking on responsibility with NASA, becoming the book review editor for the *New England Journal of Medicine*, and expressing his long-standing interest in national health policy. He also now had time to sail, and with friends became a co-owner of a forty-foot Bermuda yawl named *Angelique*. When he entered in a race and won, he served potato chips in the trophy bowl.

A new passage came when his and Laurie's youngest of five children, Chip, finished college and medical school, and was married in 1976. Franny, and his adored Laurie, then went together on medical trips. In great demand around the world, Franny took Laurie as he served as a requested speaker in England, France, Italy, Scandinavia, Australia, New Zealand, and then rounded the world through Australia, India, and China. Since Laurie had pursued her life outside of Franny's shadow studying languages and cultural history, she often became Franny's knowledgeable personal guide.

Of his long marriage he said there was no predicting a happy marriage. When one evening his children, in the midst of a vigorous argument asked, "Why did you marry Mother?" Franny instinctively shot back, "Lust." His children, despite their sophistication and growing up during the sixties sexual revolution, were shocked. Franny noted, "Children have a hard time realizing that their parents can be passionate lovers," and then listed some of the other components of a happy union: an intellectual attraction, congeniality of interests, and fidelity. At the time that his children were grilling him, he and Laurie had been married for fifty-three years. There was no way to calculate how many serious arguments they had had, he admitted, but always their double bed was a good means of conflict resolution. "You can't go to bed together if you're still mad."

On July 25, 1988, Laurie was driving home from Carlisle, northwest of Boston, near the famous town of Concord, where one of Franny's favorite authors, Ralph Waldo Emerson, had lived and written his important works in America's early days. A sudden summer thunderstorm darkened the sky and unleashed torrential rain, a storm so intense locals would remember it for years. Fifty-three years earlier, Laurie and Franny had driven through a similar storm as they began their honeymoon, and this storm seemed to be foreshadowed by that earlier one. In the downpour, Laurie could not see a loaded gravel truck bearing down on her tiny car. Franny would always describe it in a simple, emotionally laden sentence: "Laurie's life was ended in a moment of terrible encounter."

After Laurie's death, a new form of loneliness settled in. Franny reflected that, having been happily married for more than half of his life, he missed the intimacy that marriage brings. Katharyn Watson Saltonstall had been a friend of Laurie's. Franny had helped her with medical treatment for her ill husband. Like Franny, her marriage had produced a family of five children, and when her husband died, she longed for the enjoyment her family had provided her. On May 13, 1990, she and Franny married.

Their union gave Franny comfort and happiness. He said that when he heard of men who had lost their wives, or of wives who had lost their husbands, he could never wish for them a happier outcome after loneliness and grief than a marriage such as his and Katharyn's.

As Franny aged, his body turned on him; his aspirations and enjoyments could no longer be met by a physical strength he could count on. After his eightieth birthday, his days were difficult. He soldiered on for eight more years, until weakened and tortured by heart failure. He embraced his understanding from his medical school days that when the body as a dwelling place for the soul becomes no longer habitable, life had best be permitted to depart.

On November 24, 2001, Franny ended his own life.

When Charles Woods said that he did not work so hard to stay alive just to sit on his porch—or take up a home-based business of raising turkeys—he was not merely trying out words. He proved them. After starting a company to build houses during the construction boom at the end of war, he became a real estate developer, the owner of five television stations, as well as radio stations, and entered politics. He ran for governor of Alabama against George Wallace. He ran for president in 1992 against George H. Bush, which gave him a platform to speak about his populist beliefs: that America was becoming a land where the rich got richer and the poor got poorer. Remembering his childhood during the Great Depression, he longed to represent the hard-working poor.

He never won a political race, but the opportunity to be seen and heard was worth his effort. Videos are available in which he can be seen in all his scarred glory, embodying the fact that a horrendous disability is no reason to withdraw from life and public service. Often in articles, he would be described as "fire-scarred," and social media comments on his video appearances reveal the mean-spirited ignorance that the digital age has allowed to be publicly unleashed: "You almost have to admire someone that mutilated running for public office," one viewer wrote in a comment. "Or maybe pity is the word."

He spoke openly about his five years of hospitalization and the sixty operations that brought him back from certain death and gave him a face with which to walk out into the world. He would describe how the experience made him fully aware of how fragile life is. Knowing how he was forever changed by war, he emphasized that political decisions impact lives. He stated openly that before his crash, he was "self-centered and selfish. Now I am a giver instead of a taker."

For the rest of his life, he would travel to Boston for Joe to repair some damage in his scarred skin. His son David sometimes went with him. After following in his father's footsteps as a businessman, owning multiple television stations, David recalls today the times that his father sat down his six sons and three daughters asking for a complete dissertation on, *Now, why exactly are you whining?*

As for posttraumatic stress or haunting memories of the crash that could have impacted his role as a father and husband, David says he can't recall any. When Joe asked Charles to speak to Harvard Medical School students about his experiences, he always said that he was not in the least bit heroic. He stressed instead the need to keep one's head in a time of crisis. And added, "We didn't pay much attention to the decorations back then. They'd send you a certain medal for so many missions or something like that, and you'd stick it in your baggage and wouldn't give it a thought because almost never did you see anybody wearing a medal overseas. You wore your wings and your rank and that was it."

He declared that he never considered his appearance a handicap. He thought it proved useful in that no one ever forgot meeting him. It was also helpful when his competitors thought he was not very bright, so if they tried to cheat him, he relished that they thought of him enough of an equal to try to swindle him!

When he asked one of his teenaged sons what his friends thought of him (no doubt suffering at times the weight of his deformed appearance), his son answered, "They think you're magic, Daddy."

In 1990, when he heard that Joe Murray had won the Nobel Prize in Medicine and that the scientific phenomenon of his long-lasting skin grafts in 1945 had inspired Joe, he said that whenever he heard of a successful transplant, he felt a certain satisfaction. "I feel I had a small part in it, just by laying still on that table and letting Dr. Murray cut on me."

He lived a long, generous life of eighty-three years. Miriam died in 1995. Charles followed her on October 17, 2004, and is buried in Arlington National Cemetery in Washington.

In 1963, the National Academy of Sciences with the National Research Council had organized an international conference in Washington, DC, to pool and evaluate data on all human kidney transplants. Some of the best minds in the field came from France, Germany, England, Scotland, Denmark, and cities through the US. Joe chaired the meeting. Peter served in the role of premier leader in transplantation biology. By now, the cases of transplants performed around the world were staggering. Peter suggested that everyone document all past and future cases, to measure outcomes and set standards. When that program outgrew Joe's and the Brigham's ability to administer it, the government took it over and devised a worldwide system of organ procurement and distribution. That today's global kidney transplant programs function on the basis of Peter's suggestion, along with the cooperation of those few early transplant surgeons, is a fact to savor.

As Joe said of his career, using words from *Alice in Wonderland*, "It just gets curiouser and curiouser." And indeed it did, for after becoming a premier transplant surgeon who pioneered organ transplantation as an accepted form of treatment, he circled back to his interest in plastic and reconstructive surgery, first discovered at Valley Forge Hospital during the war. In 1971, he told Franny, "My heart is in reconstructive challenges, especially in children." Franny understood and shifted Joe's day-to-day coverage of transplant patients to others. Joe then gave rein to his deep-seated admiration for those struck by nature's random blow. He spent the remainder of his years as a surgeon helping mostly children whose appearance was an undeserved burden. Due to birth defects, disease, or injury, they had been turned into outcasts, vulnerable to isolation and rejection.

Joe turned to Paul Tessier, a renowned plastic surgeon from Paris who was revolutionizing the care of patients with congenital and traumatic craniofacial problems. Tessier's work was changing forever the thinking about the correction of facial deformities, and after learning the latest surgical techniques from Tessier, Joe joined him in helping to pioneer and expand the field of craniofacial surgery.

As Franny wrote, "The surgeon is never anonymous, a committee, or a corporation. Only one person makes the critical decisions and takes the crucial steps with helping hands." Of Joe he said, "Dr. Murray helped create the largest completely new field of biomedical science and clinical art to have originated entirely within this century: organ transplantation."

But always, Joe sought to be in contact with those whose courage was impervious to analysis. He cherished a letter from one of his patients, Raymond McMillan, born with deafness, a heart defect, and no control of his facial muscles, drooling constantly. Raymond's appearance was so shocking that he was even rejected by his parents and placed in an institution for the mentally disabled. After he was released at the age of twenty-one and sent out to fend for himself in the world, he wrote: "I promised myself to be so strong that nothing could disturb my peace of mind. To give so much time to the improvement of myself that I have no time to criticize another. To be too large for worry, too noble for anger, too strong for fear, and too happy to permit the presence of trouble."

Joe treasured that piece of writing. Through his skills as a surgeon, he gave Raymond the ability to smile, to speak more clearly, and to close his mouth, as well as a revised nose. His appearance, if not improved enough to blend in with ordinary humanity, was at least improved enough to give Raymond a workable life. He graduated from high school. He worked at a hospital lab in a job for which Joe helped him apply. When he died in 1997, Joe kept his writings as a cherished example of the strength of the human spirit battling adversity.

At six o'clock in the morning on March 20, 1986, Joe was getting ready to leave on an academic trip. In the shower, while mentally going over details, preparing for the days ahead, he suddenly felt a strange weakness in his left leg. Seconds later, his left arm became weak. He wished it away, but with every second, the weakness got worse. Bobby drove him straight to the Brigham, where the paralysis spread as Joe realized he was having a stroke.

As he lay in the hospital bed, he vowed that even if there would be no more hiking, tennis, mountain climbing, or other outdoor activities, he would use whatever function that remained to do what he could. He also took an inventory: the house was mortgage-free, all six children had been educated, he was due to retire anyway, and his forty-two-year career in surgery had been coming to an end.

Over the next several months, he learned to walk again. His ten-year-old grandson taught him how to throw a ball and to walk upstairs, and even ride a bicycle with no hands. In August of 1990, after he had recovered and was again puttering round his Vineyard house, he began to think that the world had passed him by. Yes, he had lived a valuable life. Yes, he had done extraordinary things and met extraordinary people, but it was all fading, not to be remembered, and he feared that his work would not be counted in a permanent inventory in the world's lists of lasting marks.

Then came the phone call.

He and Bobby were in California visiting one of their daughters.

He'd accepted an invitation to speak at the American College of Surgeons in San Francisco that October. Bobby was gently fussing because he'd forgotten to think ahead to make reservations at the San Francisco hotel where his speech would be given. Having to take the last room available, Joe humorously assumed it would be a broom closet, and he'd need to apologize to Bobby when they checked in.

The news that he had been awarded the 1990 Nobel Prize in Medicine reached his daughter Ginny in Massachusetts first; it was the middle of the night in California. An enterprising reporter hoped to be the first to deliver the news and called several San Francisco hotels, not knowing Joe was at his daughter's house. Eventually the reporter found a Dr. Murray at one of the hotels and awakened him only to find it was the wrong Murray. But Ginny knew where her father was and called her sister's number at 4:40 a.m. Only when Joe and Bobby got to their San Francisco hotel did the reality of the news really hit. The manager rushed to greet them saying that he and Bobby had been upgraded from the "broom closet" to the regency suite. Joe turned to Bobby and said, "Now I know it must be true." Bobby rolled her eyes and fondly said, "Joe Murray, you always luck out of the holes you dig for yourself!"

The whirlwind of that day never completely ended. There was a news conference and a barrage of requests for interviews. When asked if he had expected the Nobel Prize, Joe said, "I knew that I had been nominated several times over the years by a wide variety of people and groups. In 1988, the Nobel Committee had awarded the prize to my colleagues, biochemists George Hitchings and Trudy Elion, for their discoveries of important principles for drug treatment, one of which was Imuran. I interpreted this gesture as the Committee's way of acknowledging the field of transplantation and assumed they considered my transplant work to be oriented toward patient care. So I really was surprised and elated when I was notified two years later that I had been selected."

Joe was only the fourth surgeon to be given the prize; the other three were Emil Kocher of Switzerland in 1909 for his work on surgery of the thyroid gland; Alexis Carrel in 1912, the first American surgeon to be selected (although French, he was working at the Rockefeller Institute for Medical Research in New York at the time), for his technique to connect blood vessels; and Charles Huggins from the University of Chicago in 1966 for his hormonal treatment of cancer.

At the Nobel ceremony in Stockholm, Joe reveled in the quirks that stipple ordinary life. Prior to the official ceremony, the wife of a laureate fell and hurt her ankle, rather severely. Since Joe was the only clinician in the group—most being basic scientists—someone shouted, "Let's get Dr. Murray. He's the only one of us who takes care of patients for a living." No sooner was that crisis over than the next followed. On a boat trip with a group of laureates and their families, a young girl developed acute appendicitis, which Joe diagnosed, then accompanied her to a nearby hospital for her appendix to be removed before it ruptured.

Franny, wanting to relish the recognition of Joe's great achievement, traveled to Sweden to accompany him, and right before the Nobel ceremony discovered he had forgotten his pants. Making a quick visit to a tailor, he laughed when he heard the tailor yell across the room: "Well, well. Another American who forgot his trousers!"

Joe shared the Nobel Prize in Medicine with Dr. E. Donnall Thomas, who pioneered bone marrow transplantation, which saved thousands of leukemia patients.

Thanksgiving night in 2012, ninety-three-year-old Joe was savoring his long life and time with his family. Looking at the faces

249

of Bobby and his children gathered around the holiday table, no doubt he recalled the Thornton Wilder play that had reminded him throughout his life to take note of every moment and the people with whom he had shared those moments. The play had served him as a searchlight, leading the way when he needed to be guided. And as if in a perfect circular design, in the way his days had been dotted with those small things that gave his life unique meaning, he ate a piece of the chocolate pie from the same recipe as the one he had eaten on the day he asked Bobby to marry him. That night he suffered another hemorrhagic stroke and died on Monday, November 26, at Brigham and Women's Hospital, where, as a surgeon-scientist, he had pioneered the moment when borrowing organs would seem a normal, everyday way to retrieve a life.

His historic surgery was memorialized in an oil painting by Joel Babb, unveiled in 1997, to hang in the Countway Library of Harvard Medical School. Bobby lives on in the house they shared, savoring the sixty-seven years of their love affair and the knowledge that Joe continues to touch thousands of lives. Always, whenever he looked at Bobby, even after she was not only the mother of six children but also a grandmother to many, he would nod toward her and declare, "Isn't she beautiful?"

Acknowledgments

THIS BOOK TOOK its first breath on a summer day in 2017 when my husband said, "By the way, the history about Joe and the first successful human transplant of a kidney would make a mighty fine story . . ."

In May 1968, my husband graduated from Vanderbilt Medical School. That spring Dr. Francis Moore chose him to be one of eight interns in general surgery at the Brigham Hospital in Boston, with plans to train later with the eminent pediatric neurosurgeon Donald Matson.

Newly wed, we stuffed our little car with all our belongings and leapt into the future, blissfully ignorant of who Dr. Moore *really* was but enthralled with the idea of leaving the South to live in New England. When Dr. Moore learned we had no family financial support to supplement an intern's salary, he called me up and said, "I'd like to hire you to be my secretary." I can still hear his voice: kind but *so* New England, elegant and authoritative. I graciously (I hope) declined his offer, saying that I didn't have a very "secretarial nature." You see, at the age of five I decided to be a storyteller, which over the years took on the lofty goal of becoming a novelist in the good ol' southern tradition of Eudora Welty, Carson McCullers, and Faulkner. I had little patience for typing and filing, which didn't serve my creative longings. Besides, as an additional excuse, I was twenty-four and callow.

Now I am old and know better.

In those eight years of my husband's training in Boston, he also worked under Dr. Joseph Murray, doing surgical cases with him and sometimes caring for Joe's transplant patients. Five decades later, as I began researching the history of Joe's life and found its connections with the lives of Francis Moore and Peter Medawar, a story scrambled up from history and began filling blank pages. In a sense, I have finally become the secretary they all needed to step into our world. At times it seemed that while I was recreating their lives from the printed words they left, I was simply taking dictation, arousing their voices sleeping in history. And it has been my privilege to listen.

So thanks to my husband, Parker, not just for this story but for fifty-one years of adventures, to Kevin Stevens for taking on *Borrowing Life* to share with every reader lucky enough to turn the pages to get to know Joe, Franny, Peter, Charles, Jean, Miriam, Bobby, Cynthia, Ronald, and Richard. And special thanks to their families for answering the phone when I called asking for insights into the minds and work of their loved ones. Yes, Cynthia Herrick, Ronald's widow, kindly answered my phone call. As did Virginia Herrick and Van, younger sister and older brother of the Herrick twins. Also, Chip Moore, Franny's youngest son who now is a general surgeon at the Brigham; David Woods, Charles's son who has stepped into his footsteps as a TV station owner. The excitement I felt on the day I finally found a child of Charles and Miriam to help me with this story was indeed a goosebump moment. As it was when I called a Joel Babb in Maine, and he himself answered the phone saying, "Well, yes I am," when I excitedly asked, "Are you *the* Joel Babb who painted transplant history?" He has become a lifelong friend and ushered me to other sources to enrich this book, including Dr. Sukumar Desai, who wrote an article on the Babb painting that documents that historic 1954 day by showing where each participant was standing and including their signatures—a thrilling article to read, similar at looking at the signatures on the Declaration of Independence for me, and I hope for you. Publisher Mary Ann Sabia offered steadfast support as the pages of the book added up; Allison Brock made the words so much better; and Nancy Whiteman at Franny and Laurie's childhood school in Chicago, North Shore Country Day School, graciously gave us the use of photographs for this book.

A special thanks to my agent, Mark Gottlieb, who echoed my thoughts by saying he couldn't imagine this story being passed over by a publisher. To my friends, especially Vandy and Jeanne, as well as my family, who put up with my babbling about this book and being an "obsessional" in the vein of Peter Medawar. Thanks, too, to my special friend Dr. Peter Calabrese who so kindly read the final draft and kept me from making ignorant mistakes.

So go, little book, fly far and wide. Shower us with hope—what Emily Dickinson called "the thing with feathers."

Appendix

BECOMING A KIDNEY DONOR

AS OF THE PUBLICATION of this book, over a hundred thousand Americans suffering from kidney disease need a donated kidney for a transplant. On average, only seventeen thousand people each year receive a donated kidney, and every day twelve people die waiting for one. Three thousand new patients are added to the kidney waiting list each month, one every fourteen minutes.

Identifying yourself as an organ and/or tissue donor is simple. Visit the Donate Life America website (https://registerme.org/) to join your state's online registry for donation. You can also declare your intention on your driver's license. Letting your family or other loved ones know about your decision is also important. Family members are often asked to give consent for a loved one's donation, so it's important that they know your wishes.

Acceptable organ donors can range in age from newborn to sixty-five or older. Donor organs are matched to waiting recipients by a national computer registry called the National Organ Procurement and Transplantation Network. This computer registry is operated by the United Network for Organ Sharing located in Richmond, Virginia.

The NEAD, Never Ending Altruistic Donor chain, is a system founded by Garet Hill. When Hill's ten-year-old daughter developed kidney disease, he discovered he was incompatible to donate his kidney to her, so he found a cousin who was willing to donate her compatible kidney. Hill then donated one of his kidneys to a stranger, thus starting the NEAD chain, a program that matches a potential donor with a recipient who has a willing but incompatible donor.

This chain of donors has been featured in various news stories as an uplifting example of the power of individuals to affect the outcome of a debilitating disease, all stemming from the historic surgery performed by Dr. Joseph Murray on December 23, 1954.

(The above information has been compiled from the websites of the National Kidney Foundation, the NEAD™ Chain, and The National Kidney Center.)

Chronology

1912 Dr. Alexis Carrel wins the Nobel Prize for developing anastomosis, a surgical method for attaching veins and arteries and a vital technique for transplant surgery.

1913 Peter Bent Brigham Hospital in Boston opens with Dr. Harvey Cushing as Chief of Surgery.

1937 St. Louis plastic surgeon James Barrett Brown reports that skin grafts between identical twins are accepted without rejection.

1939 Peter Medawar witnesses the Spitfire crash that inspires his research into the workings of the immune system, necessary to understanding the biological forces of rejection.

1940 Survivors of the London bombings, dug from the rubble, have renal failure known as *crush syndrome*. Kept alive with blood transfusions, their kidneys often spontaneously recover, leading to the idea of dialyzing a patient to remove waste substances from the blood.

1942 Dr. Francis Moore rises to national prominence when he helps revolutionize burn care while treating victims of the Cocoanut Grove nightclub fire in Boston.

1943 The Dutch doctor Willem Kolff publishes details in a Swedish scientific journal of his invention of the first dialysis machine.

1943 With surgeon Tom Gibson, Peter Medawar publishes the discovery of the Second Set Phenomenon, also to be known as *acquired immunity*, implying that rejection is an immunological process that might be manipulated.

1944 On December 23, Charles Woods's plane crashes in India. Six weeks later he arrives at Valley Forge Military Hospital to be treated by a medical team that includes twenty-five-year-old surgeon Joseph Murray.

1946 Three doctors at the Peter Bent Brigham try a middle-of-the-night risky procedure to put a cadaver kidney in the arm of a dying woman, in the hope that it will cleanse her blood while her own kidneys heal.

1948 Dr. Hugh Donald asks Peter Medawar to come up with a foolproof method of distinguishing between fraternal and identical cattle twins, eventually leading to the ground-breaking research revealing that rejection could be subverted prior to birth.

1948 Francis Moore is named Moseley Professor of Surgery at Peter Bent Brigham a month before he turns thirty-five.

1951   Peter Medawar and Rupert "Bill" Billingham publish the first of two papers in the journal *Heredity* on the phenomenon soon to be known as *tolerance*.

1953   With Billingham and Leslie Brent, Peter Medawar publishes "Actively acquired tolerance of foreign cells" in the October 3 issue of *Nature*, the same journal in which Watson and Crick publish their work on the discovery that the genetic code for the development of an individual comes from a chemical to be known as DNA.

1954   During the summer, a team of Brigham doctors removes kidneys from recently deceased patients and attaches them to the vessels of the thighs of nine patients with kidney failure in the hope that the thigh kidneys could be a bridge for temporary function until the patients' own kidneys regain function.

1954   On December 23, Joseph Murray, with the transplant team at the Peter Bent Brigham, performs the first successful kidney transplant on identical twins Richard and Ronald Herrick.

1959   Robert Schwartz and William Dameshek, hematologists at Tufts Medical School in Boston, publish an article in *Nature* revealing the effects of the anticancer drug 6-mercaptopurine (6-MP) on the immune system. Research on the use of immunosuppressive drugs to control rejection in a transplanted kidney begins.

1959   Francis Moore, with technician Margaret Ball and medical illustrator Mildred Codding, publish *The Metabolic Care of the Surgical Patient*, one of the most widely quoted volumes in the surgical literature of the day and still in print.

1962   Transplant surgery is successfully performed on Mel Doucette, whose transplanted kidney survives with the use of immunosuppressive drugs, one of which he stays on for the rest of his life. When Doucette survives a year, Joe Murray publishes the case in the *New England Journal of Medicine*.

1963   The National Academy of Sciences/National Research Council hold an international conference in Washington, DC, to evaluate data on all human kidney transplantations to minimize errors and identify factors in donor selection and patient care that contribute to success.

Notes

These notes include material that may be of interest and have been prepared in the spirit of continuing a conversation with the reader.

A Note to Readers

"spare-parts surgery": "The ancient ambition of saving lives by means of what Murray and others have termed 'spare parts surgery'," Gösta Gahrton, in chapter 4 of *The Nobel Prize Annual, 1990*, International Merchandising Corporation (New York, 1990), 56.

"human nature in the raw": Joseph Murray, "The First Successful Organ Transplants in Man," Nobel Lecture (December 8, 1990), *Les Prix Nobel*, The Nobel Foundation 1990/1991, 202.

"Dr. Moore lives life on a different plane": Joel Babb, interview by author, February 25, 2019.

1

the largest in the United States: *Brief History of Valley Forge Hospital*, http://www.valleyforgehospital.com.

he had been drafted after Japan's attack on Pearl Harbor: Joseph Murray, *Surgery of the Soul: Reflections on a Curious Career* (Sagamore Beach, MA: Science History Publications, 2012), 28.

he was now ambidextrous: Ginny (Joe Murray's daughter), interview by author, November 10, 2017.

"Holy Joe": Eulogy for Joe Murray by his children, Ginny and Rick.

Ration cards: William Manchester, *The Glory and the Dream: A Narrative History of America 1932–1972* (Boston: Little, Brown and Company, 1974), 293.

victory gardens: Ibid., 303.

War production sent money flowing: Ibid., 280.

2

"Flying the Hump": one of the most necessary and dangerous missions in World War II: http://www.cbi-history.com/partxiihumps5.html.

a hand shaking him awake to fly the route again: John Frasca and Michael Harris, *The Sun Rose Late: The Incredible Story of Charles Woods* (Florence, AL: House of Collectibles, 1964), 6–11.

life expectancy of a World War II pilot was only thirty days: Murray, *Surgery of the Soul*, 5.

The Flying Tigers were the line of defense for the Chinese: The history of the Chinese Fighting Tigers is detailed in several sources, including the documentary *Wings Over China*. This little-known group of US pilots began as an executive order from President Roosevelt in 1940, before America entered World War II. A hundred combat pilots volunteered for the mission. They were paid for their service and were drawn from both the Army Air Corps and the navy. After Pearl Harbor, they continued their activity as part of the larger US force defending China against the Empire of Japan.

To him, Hitler was more than a funny little man: Charles Woods's feelings about Hitler's threat to the world were not common in the days when American isolationists wanted no part of the war and had no desire to come to Europe's defense. A worldwide economic depression, which had made people feel desperate to try different forms of government, had enabled totalitarianism in Germany and fascism in Italy to take control. Russia had already embraced communism. In strong language, President Roosevelt made it clear that if England fell, world totalitarianism would be emboldened and "all of us in the Americas will be living at the point of a gun" (Doris Kearns Goodwin, *No Ordinary Time: Franklin and Eleanor Roosevelt: The Home Front in World War II*, New York: Simon & Schuster, 1994, 195).

"when I was told to fly, I flew": Murray, *Surgery of the Soul*, 5.

"Maybe you weren't looking": The dialogue between Charles and Miriam when they met is from *The Sun Rose Late*, 52.

He was the only one who made it out: Ibid., 7–10. Detail and dialogue of the crash scene are from *The Sun Rose Late*. There is no record of Stalmacher's first name. However, Charles's son, Dr. Andrew M. Woods, offered the author this perspective in an email: "After my father was dead, at the end of a long life, I had the opportunity to review the accident report of his crash. In it, a night watchman reported that he saw flames erupt from one of the engines before the wing dipped and the airplane went off the runway. Thus, the loss of airspeed, and the crash, was caused by engine failure, something beyond pilot control. For his entire life, my father told the story of Stalmacher when asked 'What happened to you?'"

3

"your job is right here": Francis Moore, *A Miracle and a Privilege: Recounting a Half Century of Surgical Advance* (Washington, DC: Joseph Henry Press, 1995), 83.

cast sang some of the president's songs: Ibid., 42.

rapidly advancing field of science: Ibid., ix, 52.

automatically go to Laurie's: Ibid., 45.

4

no nose, no eyelids, no ears: Murray, *Surgery of the Soul*, 3.

between them with perfect success: Murray, *Surgery of the Soul*, 69, and Moore, *A Miracle and a Privilege*, 171.

2.3 million doses of penicillin to be produced in time for the invasion of Normandy: internet research on penicillin and Francis Moore's description of caring for patients in the Cocoanut Grove fire when so few doses were available.

The trip had taken six agonizing weeks: The description of Charles Woods's trip to Valley Forge is from *The Sun Rose Late*, 35–66.

5

feet were too big: Peter Medawar, *Memoir of a Thinking Radish: An Autobiography* [a blend of Pascal's term "a thinking reed" and Shakespeare's character Falstaff's comment, "forked radish"] (Oxford: Oxford University Press, 1986), 74.

leftover ether: Jean Medawar, *A Very Decided Preference: Life with Peter Medawar* (New York: W. W. Norton & Company, 1990), 65.

"take a serious interest in real life": Medawar, *Memoir of a Thinking Radish*, 22.

between *self* and *non-self*: Medawar, *A Very Decided Preference*, 52.

"fritter away my time": Medawar, *Memoir of a Thinking Radish*, 77.

"messings about": Ibid.

not gotten off the ground: Ibid., 63.

"saffron as a microscopic stain": Ibid., 59.

burned pilot died of infection: Nicholas L. Tilney, *Transplant: From Myth to Reality* (New Haven: Yale University Press, 2003), 109. In contrast to Jean and Peter Medawar's memoirs, which state the pilot most likely lived. Jean thought she heard he had relocated to Canada.

"pleasure to investigate": Medawar, *Memoir of a Thinking Radish*, 78.

"where Peter got his IQ": John Maynard Smith interview, YouTube, https://youtu.be/15/sc_M322M.

summons his student for an interview: Ibid., 49.

"demography and ecology": Medawar, *Memoir of a Thinking Radish*, 54.

"move in different circles": Ibid., 182.

"mildly diabolical": Medawar, *A Very Decided Preference*, 19.

"Because it's all in the textbooks": Ibid., 20.

"He's got Arab blood": Ibid.

"the human predicament": Medawar, *Memoir of a Thinking Radish*, Introduction.

"rich tapestry of life": Medawar, *A Very Decided Preference*, 238.

"everyone saw it": Ibid., 22.

6

Joe Murray's response to witnessing Charles Woods's long-lasting cadaver "borrowed" skin grafts, known as allografts, is drawn from his description in *Surgery of the Soul*, 9.

"a charm to wean us": Tilney, *Transplant*, 30.

small molecules passed through: Moore, *A Miracle and a Privilege*, 168.

Blood transfusions had been found to be the prime treatment for shock: Steven R. Pierce, "Blood Transfusion in the First World War," in *Medicine in the First World War*, http://www.kumc.edu/wwi/essays-on-first-world-war-medicine/index-of-essays/medicine.html; also available in Tilney, *Transplant*, 20. Using blood as a treatment to restore health was first evidenced in the seventeenth-century practice of bloodletting, known as *venesection*. After William Harvey in England described the circulation of blood in 1628, he suggested injecting fluids into the bloodstream. Shortly after, the famous architect Christopher Wren performed intravenous injections in dogs. Several disastrous attempts to inject animal blood into humans led to blood transfusions being forbidden in France. At the beginning of the eighteenth century, Karl Landsteiner discovered the differences of A, B, and O blood groups, which then led physicians to realize that blood transfusions between the groups caused inflammation and clumping of red blood, and that donor serum and recipient cells *must* be matched. Over the centuries, transfusions became common and the technology of storing blood improved to the point where blood could be stored in large enough quantities for use in wartime. By World War II, storing blood was a common practice, and the Red Cross set up blood banks throughout Europe. Ironically, while all backgrounds and classes of soldiers—rich, poor, those of Italian or Irish heritage, those from the Midwest, East, the South—mingled in the effort to win World War II, the blood of different races was not allowed to be mingled. Racist attitudes were so entrenched that stored blood to treat injured African-American soldiers was kept separate from blood to be used in transfusions for white soldiers (Manchester, *The Glory and the Dream*, 283).

7

The chapter title quote is from Manchester's *The Glory and the Dream*, 363.

Charles's America was changing: Drawn from Manchester's *The Glory and the Dream*, 290, and Kearns Goodwin, *No Ordinary Time*, 450.

able to pen his signature: as noted by Daisy Suckley in Geoffrey Ward, ed., *Closest Companion: The Unknown Story of the Intimate Friendship between Franklin Roosevelt and Margaret Suckley* (New York: Simon & Schuster, 1995), 326.

cost the lives: The estimate of lives lost if Japan were invaded to end the war comes from Jean Edward Smith's *FDR* (New York: Random House, 2007), 629.

Since October 1939: Detail about the making of the atom bomb, the letter to Einstein, FDR's reaction is from Manchester's *The Glory and the Dream*, 210–16. The link between the splitting of the atom and the irradiation of patients and bone marrow transfusions to depress the immune system, as well as the government's encouragement to find treatments for survivors of nuclear war, comes from Moore's explanation in *Give and Take: The Biology of Tissue Transplantation* (New York: Anchor Books, 1965), in which he wrote: "The sort of treatment being given here, after the irradiation dosage, had been under close study in several laboratories since World War II, because it is the sort of treatment that might be used for survivors of an atomic bomb explosion such as that which occurred at Hiroshima and Nagasaki. It was well known that bone-marrow transfusions might be an important treatment during a nuclear war. Here was a patient [Gladys Loman] who had received a lethal amount of radiation to the whole body. Damage was severe, not only to the antibody-forming cells, but also to those components of blood that make it clot" (102).

"You have first claim on my love": Medawar, *A Very Decided Preference*, 39. Jean's adjustment to Peter's restless mind and his ignoring her, to which in time she learned to ask, "Are you thinking?" as well as the description of their marriage and commitment to each other is drawn from her memoir, *A Very Decided Preference*, 15–40.

burns unit of Glasgow Royal Infirmary: Ibid., 53.

foreign grafts from a close relative: Ibid., 54.

a sign of inflammation: Medawar, *A Memoir of a Thinking Radish*, 82.

then couldn't it be potentially manipulated?: Ibid, 53.

"The Fate of Skin Homografts in Man": Medawar, *A Memoir of a Thinking Radish*, 82.

Joe noted that: Murray, "The First Successful Organ Transplant in Man," 205.

no trained technicians to call upon: Ibid., 83.

8

"The rest is all decorations": Frasca and Harris, *The Sun Rose Late*, 80.

He asked a nurse for a hand mirror: Ibid., 85, 102–103.

and looked in the mirror there: Charles Woods's reaction to seeing his reconstructed face and his response to realizing he is not blind is drawn from *The Sun Rose Late*, 84–85. His resilience might be illuminated by the study that forty years later author and editor Norman Cousins undertook for what he called "the biology of hope." Finding that patients who set goals for themselves dealt better with a physical challenge, he also conducted studies to see if the immune system strengthens from having a positive outlook. He witnessed that humor and laughing allowed patients to tolerate pain. Studies have shown that the brain can order the release of secretions, known as endorphins and enkephalins, to act as the body's own painkillers. In a 2013 article in

Neuroscience, five researchers stated that morphine as an analgesic compound for pain relief is synthesized by mammalian cells from dopamine, the chemical in the brain that acts as a messenger, sending signals from one nerve cell to another and connecting the brain with its reward and pleasure centers. Furthermore, Charles had goals, including returning to Alabama and supporting Miriam and Freddie. No doubt, too, he had what would become known as "survivors' guilt." How he would deal with those emotional scars after his release from the Valley Forge Hospital was yet to be seen, although his son David told the author there were no signs of PTSD that he ever witnessed in his father. Charles Woods was a testament to what research would later find out, as Norman Cousins put it in his 1989 *Head First: The Biology of Hope and Healing Power* (New York: Penguin Books), "for those facing physical adversity life was the ultimate prize. Those who fought to survive discovered how tentative and fragile life can be, and that the essential art of living is to recognize and savor the preciousness of each minute when it is free of imminent threat or jeopardy" (107).

drink it straight up: Joe Murray's love of chocolate syrup was detailed in an email interview with his son Rick in September 2017. The description of his proposal to Bobby comes from *Surgery of the Soul,* 43–44.

9

"Give as much motion as possible": Murray, *Surgery of the Soul,* 12.

"We're calling her the *poetry lady*": Fresca and Harris, *The Sun Rose Late,* 102–103.

To duplicate his findings of the second set phenomenon: Medawar, *Memoir of a Thinking Radish,* 86. Illuminating Peter Medawar's research on the second set phenomenon, Moore, in *Give and Take,* 22–23, discussed Medawar's pointing to an old study from 1923, performed by a young surgical resident at Johns Hopkins, Emile Holman. Dr. Holman did skin grafts on a five-year-old boy whose leg had been mangled. Since his mother's blood was compatible, Dr. Holman took 151 pinch grafts from her thigh and put them onto part of her son's wound. Seven days later he took 168 additional pinch grafts from her and grafted them onto the rest of her son's leg. At first all the grafts seemed to be taking. But about two weeks after the second skin graft, the boy developed severe inflammation all over his skin with itching and peeling. His skin also had marked desiccation (drying out) "on his scalp, face, arms and legs." Dr. Holman soon decided that the general dermatitis was most probably a phenomenon of anaphylaxis (heightened immunity) or protein intoxication; the boy was sensitive to the foreign protein of his mother. He decided to take an all-important step, to wait three and a half months and remove all the skin grafts. Soon the dermatitis rapidly disappeared. This was the first patient known to be sensitized by his mother's skin, evidenced by an inflammation of his own tissues. In other words, he became allergic to his mother's skin, and his body's quick reaction to his mother's foreign protein ignited his immune system to be inflamed even to his own tissues, to attack skin on his scalp as if it were foreign, a phenomenon that today might be referred to as an autoimmune disease like multiple sclerosis and rheumatoid arthritis. To expand this knowledge, Dr. Holman began a study on a twenty-eight-month-old child who had been burned on her face and body. This time a third donor was used. He took twelve pinches of skin from two different donors and nine from a third donor. At first, all the grafts seemed to be thriving and spreading. Then, at different times, from five days to a week, the grafts were rejected and disappeared. And each did so on its own schedule of rejection. The immune process was now seen clearly at work. Each group of grafts had developed its own warlike antibody to fight the new skin. But the exact mechanism for how the young child's body recognized foreign material and reacted to it as dangerous was still a mystery. Forty years later, thinking back on his experiments, Dr. Holman wrote in a letter, "What an opportunity we missed by not pursuing this further!"

his work seemed a picnic: Medawar, *Memoir of a Thinking Radish*, 86.

medical needs in Europe: Ibid., 82–84.

"a new relationship to the universe": Manchester, *The Glory and the Dream*, 275. Eight days after "the gadget" was tested, President Truman approved strikes on Hiroshima, Kokura, Niigata, and Nagasaki. As the decision looked cold-blooded, he and his secretary of war agreed there must be a "last-chance warning" given to Tokyo. The target sites were soon revised to Nagasaki and Hiroshima because of weather and the distance from B-29 bases in the Mariana Islands.

The war that had killed: The National Archives, "Pieces of History," https://prologue.blogs.archives.gov/.

10

"You were no raving beauty": Frasca and Harris, *The Sun Rose Late*, 100.

"How y'all doing?": Ibid., 111.

"God didn't give me back my life": Charles Woods's adjustment to life after Valley Forge Hospital is drawn from *The Sun Rose Late*, 153–155.

11

then commanded, "Discuss!": Medawar, *A Very Decided Preference*, 62.

left a blueprint: Moore, *A Miracle and a Privilege*, 253.

"It will never work": Murray, *Surgery of the Soul*, 63.

"a bunch of fools": Ibid., 62.

no real importance to Americans: Ibid., 23.

"So I can't be too bad": Murray, *Surgery of the Soul*, 24.

"days are too short": Ibid., 27.

medical practice and training changed: Moore, *A Miracle and a Privilege*, 13.

"Now you tie the cord": Ibid.

"Alright, Moorie": Ibid., 9.

Franny had always interpreted: Ibid., 6.

"I am a soul, I live in a body": Ibid., 5.

"Injury and disease": Ibid., 5.

"develop skin of exactly the right thickness": Ibid., 70.

he thought her death was his fault: Ibid., 68–69.

"When the anesthetist lovingly": Ibid., 72.

"the chemistry of getting well": Ibid., 109.

"I led a whirlwind existence": Ibid., 85.

"Here comes the Mose": J. P. Mickle, interview by author.

a list led by Harvey Cushing: Murray, *Surgery of the Soul*, 233.

12

"You'll need some help": Frasca and Harris, *The Sun Rose Late*, 140–149.

going over and over: Murray, *Surgery of the Soul*, 48.

she was moments from death: Moore, *A Miracle and a Privilege*, 164.

One so desperate to live: Tilney, *Transplant*, 41.

his dark side: Rebecca Skloot, *The Immortal Life of Henrietta Lacks* (New York: Crown Publishing Group, 2010), 60–61.

Soon, she walked out: This dramatic account of a cadaver kidney being placed in a twenty-nine-year-old woman's arm to rescue her from renal shutdown is described in Murray's Nobel lecture and expanded in Moore's *Give and Take*, 16–17, and *A Miracle and a Privilege*, 164–166. Murray cites R. J. Glaser's "Footnotes to Kidney Transplant History," (news release, March 31, 1988, Harvard University News Office of the Medical Area, Boston). "Dr. Glaser, assistant resident on the medical service at the time stated 'secretion of urine was minimal, and certainly did not rescue the woman from her crisis. The kidney functioned poorly and the patient continued to have a stormy course, although fortunately, despite our lack of understanding at the time of how best to treat renal shutdown, she ultimately did respond and she left the hospital with normal renal function in good health. She died a few months later of fulminating hepatitis secondary to pooled plasma infusions which she had received in the course of her treatment'."

13

Dating back to his Oxford days: Peter Medawar's meeting C. S. Lewis and T. S. Eliot is drawn from *Memoir of a Thinking Radish*, 88–89.

If they last indefinitely: Medawar's meeting with Scottish veterinarian Dr. Hugh Donald comes from his memoir, 110–112, and Jean Medawar's memoir, 67–68.

To help himself understand: Tilney, *Transplant*, 114.

"the things that generate antagonism": Moore, *Give and Take*, 25.

studies at Stanford: Tilney, *Transplant*, 114.

Perhaps the best illustration: David M. Oshinsky, *Polio: An American Story* (New York: Oxford University Press, 2005), 119.

many began to think of animals: Tilney, *Transplant*, 122–124.

"olives around his table": Medawar, *A Very Decided Preference*, 48.

Going down the alphabet: Ibid., 79.

14

"How about": Murray, *Surgery of the Soul*, 60.

"Let me take a look": John Shillito Jr., "Donald Darrow Matson, 1913–1969," *Journal of Neurological Surgery* 20 (1983), 437–39.

hope to those: Moore, *Give and Take*, 70–71.

"a start must be made": Ibid., 72.

15

Jean was worried: Jean Medawar's description of their move to London comes from *A Very Decided Preference*, 75–76.

By duplicating Hašek's findings: Medawar, *Memoir of a Thinking Radish*, 133.

a discovery that applied: Tilney, *Transplant*, 42.

"not a good moment": Medawar, *Memoir of a Thinking Radish*, 117.

"if I were to do it": Ibid.

Peter rushed her: Medawar, *A Very Decided Preference*, 70–71.

Scientists were crying out: Tilney, *Transplant*, 118.

"born anew": Medawar, *Memoir of a Thinking Radish*, 179.

"My mind, you know...or anyone else": Medawar, *A Very Decided Preference*, 47.

His standards were: Medawar, *Memoir of a Thinking Radish*, 7.

"Well, you can't please everybody": Ibid., 34.

wedding ring left imprints: Medawar, *A Very Decided Preference*, 43.

16

In 1948, the organizers: The cultural changes in the 1950s come from Manchester's *The Glory and the Dream*, 585–586.

Peter and Billingham: Medawar, *A Very Decided Preference*, 67–68.

"about 1950, some French workers": Moore, *Give and Take*, 110.

"must remain a mystery": Ibid., 75.

"the degree of the genetic disparity": The case of the first kidney transplanted from another, living for 175 days, comes from Murray's Nobel lecture and Moore's *Give and Take*, 74.

Franny took note of a curious case: Moore, *Give and Take*, 82.

In 1951, Peter and Billingham: The date of Peter's first publication on his cattle twin research in the journal *Heredity* is documented as 1950 on the internet. Peter notes the publication as 1951 in *Memoir of a Thinking Radish*, 112.

Each morning, Joe ate: Interview with Ginny Murray, November 2017, and Rick Murray, email message to author.

"By the way, this patient has an identical twin": The description of the phone call referring Richard Herrick to Joe Murray comes from Murray's *Surgery of the Soul*; Moore's *Give and Take* and *A Miracle and a Privilege*; Tilney's *Transplant*; as well as *Time Magazine*, May 3, 1963, p. 60.

17

easy way to tell the twins apart: Family stories, details, and dialogue for this chapter came from interviews with Ronald and Richard's younger sister, Virginia, and Ronald's widow, Cynthia Herrick, as well as an article written by their aunt, Virginia S. Herrick: "He Gave His Kidney to His Brother," *The Saturday Evening Post*, November 19, 1955.

How beautifully they sang: Cynthia Herrick, *The Best He Had to Offer: The Ron Herrick Story* (self-published, Cynthia Herrick, 2004): The story of her marriage to Ronald and the gift of his kidney to his brother.

"We knew he wasn't going to make it": Murray, *Surgery of the Soul*, 75.

"This other brother is a twin": Herrick, "He Gave His Kidney."

18

Dr. Francis Moore, in *Give and Take, The Biology of Tissue Transplantation*, acknowledged those who played a part in the first successful organ transplant, as well as in the eventual success in breeching the rejection barrier by immunosuppression drugs: Dr. John Merrill and Dr. J. Hartwell Harrison took responsibility for medical care and kidney-donor management as well as giving guidance of broad policy. Dr. George Thorn, Hersey Professor and physician-in-chief, helped perfect the artificial kidney following Kolff's blueprints. Others playing significant parts were: Dr. John Brooks, Dr. Richard Wilson, Dr. David Hume, Dr. Edward Hager, Dr. Somers Sturgis, Dr. Dwight Harken, Dr. Donald Matson, Dr. Nathan Couch, Dr. Ben Miller, Dr. Warren Guild, Dr. Frank Takacs, Dr. Charles Carpenter, Dr. J. M. Corson, Dr. John Luck, as well as Dr. Gustave Dammin (pathologist-in-chief) and Dr. James Dealy Jr. (radiologist-in-chief). Funding sources were Harvard University, the Peter Bent Brigham Hospital, the Avalon Foundation, the Hartford Foundation, the Strasburger Foundation, the Atomic Energy Commission, the United States Army, and the National Institutes of Health.

"When seen on October 27 and 28th": Murray, *Surgery of the Soul*, 74.

"a tremendous shot in the arm": Ibid., 86.

Blood tests: Tilney, *Transplant*, 57.

What did not occur to him: Murray, *Surgery of the Soul*, 74.

"We have to be careful": Ibid., 76–78.

Pity for the sick brother: Herrick, "He Gave His Kidney."

"Think long and hard about it": The conversation among family members with Ronald Herrick and physicians at the Brigham comes from Virginia Herrick, "He Gave His Kidney," and Cynthia Herrick, *The Best He Had to Offer.*

Weighing most heavily on Joe: Murray, *Surgery of the Soul*, 77–78.

19

While planning the surgery: Murray, *Surgery of the Soul*, 82.

A test run: Ibid., 79–83.

"Let things stand": Herrick, "He Gave His Kidney," 158.

Coordinating the timing: Murray, *Surgery of the Soul*, 79.

At the Murray house: Murray, *Surgery of the Soul*, 86, and interview with Ginny Murray, November 7, 2017.

widespread public interest: Tilney, *Transplant*, 62.

risky surgery: Ibid.

all the radios: Murray, *Surgery of the Soul*, 80.

"wordless prayer": Ibid.

he lifted out the donated kidney: Tilney, *Transplant*, 62.

The surgery was set: Murray, *Surgery of the Soul*, 80–82.

Within days: Moore, *A Miracle and a Privilege*, 173.

On January 29, 1955, Joe wrote: Murray, *Surgery of the Soul*, 83–85.

He deferred credit: "A Brother's Love Saves a Life, Makes History," USATODAY. com, December 19, 2004.

Richard would later admit: Betty Lilyestrom, "Twin Who Got Kidney Won Nurse's Heart Too," *Worcester Telegram*, 1955.

20

Over the next four years: Moore, *Give and Take*, 87.

he had practiced on dogs: Tilney, *Transplant*, 20.

Sixty years later: Marcus du Sautoy, *The Great Unknown: Seven Journeys to the Frontiers of Science* (New York: Viking, 2016), 9.

"If a line of red blood cells": Moore, *Give and Take*, 3–4. The general description of the working of the immune system comes from *Give and Take*, which Dr. Moore first prepared as a lecture in 1960 to his Harvard College Class of 1935 to tell the story of transplantation when the lay public was hungry to learn about this new universe. Dr. Moore and Dr. Murray presented a clinic on organ transplantation for this audience of nearly a thousand. The book *Give and Take*, published in 1965, grew from that lecture.

research, performed years before: Joe Murray's decision to use bone marrow transfusions comes from his memoir, *Surgery of the Soul*, 94, referencing his idea from the bone marrow research of Dr. E. Donnall Thomas, who would share the 1990 Nobel Prize in Medicine.

It was a trick that Franny liked: Moore, *Give and Take*, 95.

21

She recognized: Jean Medawar's searching for a life outside of Peter's shadow is drawn from *A Very Decided Preference*, 82–88.

He said that a fellow obsessional: Medawar, *Memoir of a Thinking Radish*, 150.

To my darling wife: Medawar, *A Very Decided Preference*, 89.

"The intensity of scientific interest": Moore, *Give and Take*, 44.

"as though supercharged": Medawar, *A Very Decided Preference*, 95.

"I don't think I should be": Ibid., 101.

"those who shall have conferred": Stig Ramel, President at the Nobel Foundation, "Introduction," The Nobel Prize Annual, 1990, XII.

"I have a very decided preference": Medawar, *A Very Decided Preference*, 10.

22

"Romance was": Manchester, *The Glory and the Dream*, 853.

Dr. Hašek, filling the house: Murray, *Surgery of the Soul*, 235.

his love for Bobby: Interview with Ginny Murray, November 2017.

Now as Joe asked Don: Murray, *Surgery of the Soul*, 95.

"the balance of survival had tipped": Moore, *Give and Take*, 103.

"vain effort to save her life": Moore, *A Miracle and a Privilege*, 176.

"There is a crack in everything": Moore, *Give and Take*, 113.

"We came so close": Murray, *Surgery of the Soul*, 96.

23

Franny was worried: Joe Murray's response to so many failures comes from the chapter "One Month in the Big House," *Surgery of the Soul*, 96–97.

"Cremation ain't so bad": Rick Murray in his eulogy for his father, December 1, 2012.

He took heart: Murray, *Surgery of the Soul*, 226.

A twelve-year-old Swedish boy: Moore, *Give and Take*, 104.

"the balance of survival": Ibid., 105.

He even went so far: Tilney, *Transplant*, 72.

24

He preferred remaining: Tilney, *Transplant*, 151.

And it started with John Riteris: The case of the Riteris brothers comes from Murray's *Surgery of the Soul*, in the chapter "John Riteris, First Allogenic (Non-identical Twins) Kidney Transplant," 99–103. Moore, in *A Miracle and a Privilege*, 170–171, points out: "In the western European races, twinning occurs about once in 85 to 90 births. Identical twinning occurs in humans about once in every 250 to 270 births, so one-third of all twins are identical. Most twins are fraternal, meaning two eggs are fertilized simultaneously by two sperm and are implanted at two different sites in the lining of the uterus to form two separate embryos with two distinct placentas that grow close together. Hence the term *fraternal twin*, meaning sibling twins. They won't look too much alike and are immunologically distinctive individuals and can be of opposite sexes. However, in identical human twins, one egg is fertilized by one sperm and then splits into two embryos that share a single placenta. Fraternal twinning is an inherited trait while identical twinning does not seem to have a genetic or familial connection, but is possibly only by chance. Identical twinning happens in all races and ethnic groups but at differing frequencies in different animals." In *Surgery of the Soul*, p. 68, Murray comments on an eerie coincidence arising from his study of classical painting. "By a remarkable stroke of luck, an opportunity [to transplant a kidney from an identical twin to bypass rejection] presented itself. Even more remarkably, years later I discovered a somewhat prophetic event in Christian hagiography. In the 4th-century Saints Cosmas and Damian, twin brothers, transplanted a limb from a black prisoner to a white recipient—an event portrayed in a number of classic paintings. I have examined such paintings in museums and galleries all over the world, and Cosmas and Damian are always depicted as identical twins." The irony that the surgeons were the identical twins rather than the transplant patients is intriguing, as if the painting was planting a subconscious hint for science to discover centuries later.

"It was one of the most critical": Moore, *Give and Take*, 108.

John Riteris was the first human: Murray, *Surgery of the Soul*, 100.

a group in Paris confirmed: Tilney, *Transplant*, 73.

"like hitting the jackpot": Moore, *Give and Take*, 110.

Andrew downplayed: Murray, *Surgery of the Soul*, 100.

25

a better protocol: Discovering the use of immunosuppressive drugs is drawn from Murray's *Surgery of the Soul*, 109, and Moore's *Give and Take*, 130–131.

Honest John: Moore, *Give and Take*, photo inset, plate 7, "Honest John."

healthy puppies, Ibid., plate 9b.

Donald Toby was only twenty-two: The case of Donald Toby comes from Murray's *Surgery of the Soul*, 113–114.

26

So for Mel: The case of Mel Doucette comes from Murray's *Surgery of the Soul*, 115–117.

From the days when Kolff: The complications that Mel Doucette faced come from Moore, *Give and Take*, 135–140.

Over the next three decades: Murray's Nobel lecture, 211.

Furthermore, the article pointed out: "Surgery: the Best Hope of All," *Time Magazine*, Henry R. Luce, Editor, Gilbert Cant, Medical Editor, May 3, 1963, Vol. LXXXI, No. 18, 57–60.

"Spare parts may be available": Ibid.

"unwanted prominence": Franny Moore's response to the *Time Magazine* article comes from his memoir *A Miracle and a Privilege*, 310.

With the assassination: Ibid., 311.

Joe would say: Murray, "The First Successful Organ Transplant in Man," 203.

"Here I was": Moore, *A Miracle and a Privilege*, "Introduction."

It was a good time: Murray, *Surgery of the Soul*, 110, and Medawar, *Memoir of a Thinking Radish*, 135.

EPILOGUE

The last normal day: The details of Peter's stroke are detailed in Jean Medawar's memoir, *A Very Decided Preference*, 13–18. His death, 241.

Soon after Ronald Herrick: Cynthia Herrick, email interview and her book, *The Best He Had to Offer*, 13, 42.

In 1984, he committed suicide: Tilney, *Transplant*, 115, and Murray, *Surgery of the Soul*, 234. Although Hašek's suicide is not included in biographical material about him on the internet, both Tilney and Murray include it in their books. Joe Murray writes in the chapter notes of *Surgery of the Soul* (234): "Sadly Milan and his wife, Vera, who was also a transplantation immunologist, were not allowed to travel together to the United States, and political constraints in the Soviet Union hindered their further progress in the field. I was saddened to hear of Milan's suicide in 1984. The affection and esteem in which he was held by his students and colleagues resulted in a memorial volume called *Realm of Tolerance*."

Don jokingly replied: Murray, *Surgery of the Soul*, 95, and J. Parker Mickle, MD, who, as a Brigham intern, helped in the care of Don Matson when he was dying.

By 1972, he was tired: Moore, *A Miracle and Privilege*, 346. Franny's life with Laurie, 47–48, her death, 351.

When Charles Woods said: Charles's adjustment to life after Valley Forge comes from Frasca and Harris, *The Sun Rose Late*, 155–156, and phone conversations as well as emails with David Woods, his son, summer 2018, adding to Joseph Murray's descriptions of Charles talking to medical students at the Brigham, *Surgery of the Soul*, 14, 227.

The government took over: Joe Murray's description of a national kidney registry and the business side of transplantation come from his memoir *Surgery of the Soul*, 120.

As Joe said of his career: Joe's dedicating the remainder of his professional life to craniofacial reconstructive surgery comes from his *Surgery of the Soul*, 162–163.

Franny understood: Francis Moore's assessment of Joe Murray's contribution to medicine comes from his preface to *Surgery of the Soul*, xxi, xxiii.

"I promised myself": Raymond McMillan's letter is in *Surgery of the Soul*, 228.

Thanksgiving night in 2012: Details from Joe's last piece of chocolate pie were provided by Joe's son, Rick Murray, in an interview with the author.

Bibliography

"A Brother's Love Saves a Life, Makes History." USATODAY.com (December 19, 2004).

Cousins, Norman. *Head First: The Biology of Hope and the Healing Power of the Human Spirit.* New York: Penguin Books, 1990.

Du Sautoy, Marcus. *The Great Unknown: Seven Journeys to the Frontiers of Science.* New York: Viking, 2017.

Evans, Harold. *The American Century.* New York: Knopf, 1998.

"Flying the Hump." http://www.cbi-history.com/part_xii_hump5.html.

Frasca, John, and Harris, Michael. *The Sun Rose Late: The Incredible Story of Charles Woods.* Florence, Alabama: House of Collectibles, 1974.

Goodwin, Doris Kearns. *No Ordinary Time.* New York: Simon and Schuster, 1995.

Herrick, Cynthia B. *The Best He Had to Offer.* Rockland, Maine: self-published, 2004.

Herrick, Virginia S. "He Gave His Kidney To His Brother." *The Saturday Evening Post* (November 19, 1955).

"Herrick Twins: Reconstructing Lives." Center for the History of Medicine Digital Collection. http://collections.countway.harvard.edu/onview/exhibits/show/reconstructing-lives/transplantion 6/1/2017.

Lilyestrom, Betty. "Twin who Got Kidney Won Nurse's Heart Too." *Worcester Telegram* (undated clipping, 1955).

Manchester, William. *The Glory and the Dream: A Narrative History of America, 1932-1972.* Boston: Little, Brown, 1973, 1974.

Marrin, Albert, *Stalin: Russia's Man of Steel.* New York: Viking Penguin, 1988.

Medawar, Jean. *A Very Decided Preference: Life with Peter Medawar.* New York, London: Norton, 1990.

Medawar, Peter. *Memoir of a Thinking Radish: An Autobiography.* Oxford: Oxford University Press, 1986.

Moore, Francis D., MD. *Give and Take: The Biology of Tissue Transplantation.* New York: Doubleday, 1965.

_____ *A Miracle and a Privilege: Recounting a Half Century of Surgical Advance.* Washington, DC: Joseph Henry Press, 1995.

Murray, Joseph E. *Surgery of the Soul, Reflections on a Curious Career.* Sagamore Beach, Massachusetts: Science History Publications, 2012.

_____ "The First Successful Organ Transplant in Man." Nobel address, The Nobel Foundation, 1991.

Noonan, Peggy. *When Character Was King: A Story of Ronald Reagan.* New York: Penguin Books, 2001.

"Organ Transplants: A Brief History." www.history.com/news/organ-transplants-a-brief-history.

Porter, Roy, ed. *The Cambridge History of Medicine.* Cambridge: Cambridge University Press, 2006.

Schlesinger, Arthur M. Jr. *A Life in the 20th Century: Innocent Beginnings, 1917-1950.* Boston, New York: Houghton Mifflin, 2000.

John Shillito Jr., MD. "Donald Darrow Matson, 1913-1969." *Journal of Neurological Surgery,* No. 20 (1983): 437-39.

Sifferlin, Alexandra. "How the First Successful Kidney Transplant Happened." TIME.com (December 23, 2014).

Skloot, Rebecca. *The Immortal Life of Henrietta Lacks.* New York: Random House, 2016.

Smith, Jean Edward. *FDR.* New York: Random House, 2007.

"Surgery: the Best Hope of All." *Time Magazine,* Vol. LXXXI, No. 18 (May 3, 1963): 57–60.

Tilney, Nicholas L., MD. *Transplant: From Myth to Reality.* New Haven and London: Yale University Press, 2003.

Ward, Geoffrey C., ed. *Closest Companion: The Unknown Story of the Intimate Friendship Between Franklin Roosevelt and Margaret Suckley.* New York: Simon and Schuster, 1995.

Photograph List and Credits

Grateful acknowledgment is made for permission to reproduce the following:

Frontispiece: *Soldiers being transported by train to the Valley Forge Military Hospital, 15 May, 1943; Philadelphia Record photograph morgue [V07]*: image courtesy of the Historical Society of Pennsylvania

Portrait of Dr. Joseph Edward Murray: image courtesy of the Archives of the American College of Surgeons

Portrait of Dr. Francis Daniels Moore: image courtesy of the Archives of the American College of Surgeons

Sir Peter Brian Medawar at his microscope: Getty/Corbis Historical

Joe and Bobby Murray in Atlantic City: image courtesy of the Murray family

Jean and Peter Medawar: file photo by United Press International

Miriam and Charles Woods: image courtesy of David D. Woods

Laurie and Franny Moore: image courtesy of North Shore Country Day School

Charles Woods campaigning: AP Photo

Charles Woods in uniform: image courtesy of David D. Woods

Cocoanut Grove nightclub fire: Getty/Bettmann

Herrick twins leaving the hospital: AP Photo/File

Ronald Herrick and nurse: Getty/Bettmann

Painting of "The First Successful Kidney Transplantation," by Joel Babb (oil on linen, hanging in the Countway Library of Medicine, Harvard Medical School): image courtesy of Joel Babb

Key to Babb painting and signatures: from the article "A Semi-Centennial Report on the Participants Depicted in Joel Babb's Portrait, 'The First Successful Kidney Transplantation',," by S. P. Desai et al; reproduced courtesy of Sukumar P. Desai

Joe Murray showing his Nobel citation: Getty/Boston Globe

Bobby and Joe Murray seated on couch: image courtesy of the Murray family/Elena Nuciforo

Index

6-MP, 217–18, 256

A

actinomycin, 223–24
Addison, Joseph, 128
allografts, 28, 30, 39–40, 42, 259
American College of Surgeons, 248
anaphylaxis, 261
anesthesia
    administered, 111–12
    local, 64, 117, 134
animal models, 118, 127–29, 139, 149, 174
antibodies, 125, 150–51, 186–88, 217, 225
Arnold Arboretum, the, 67
artificial kidney. *See* kidneys, artificial
Austen, Jane, 123
autografts, 28
azathioprine, 219

B

Babb, Joel, 250, 252
Bacon, Sir Francis, 233
bacteria, 29, 60, 133, 187
Ball, Margaret R., 111, 256
Billingham, Bill, 124, 137
blood corpuscles, 125
blood count, 208
blood pressure, 117, 181, 225
    high, 147, 159
blood pump, 119
blood tests, 166, 265
blood transfusion theory, 184
body X ray, total, 209
Bohr, Niels, 54
bone marrow, 188, 202, 208, 217, 220
bone marrow infusions, 200, 209, 218
Boston Children's Hospital, 114, 132, 135
Boylston Medical Society, 99
Bright, Richard, 94
Bright's disease, 94, 151, 157, 160
Brigham Hospital, 67, 111, 251, 255
    and Harvard Medical School, 210
    commitment to renal research and
        innovation, 93

    lab, 129
    pathology department, 175
    reputation, 93
    surgeons, 163
    transplant team, 134, 146, 151–52, 168,
        171–72, 175, 183, 185–88, 200
Brighton Marine Hospital, 151, 160–61
Burnet, Frank, 125

C

cadaver allografts, 50
cadaver kidney, 117, 120–21, 165, 222, 255, 263
cadaver skin grafts, 40
Cannon, Bradford, 131–32, 205
cardiac irregularities, 175
Carrel, Alexis, 118–20, 134, 249, 255
cattle, 76, 98, 164, 238
cells
    antibody-forming, 260
    antibody-producing, 202
    cultivated, 34
    exchanged, 184
    foreign, 138, 147, 256
    interchanged, 184
    invade, 60
    mammalian, 261
Chaplin, Charlie, 194
Cocoanut Grove fire, 24–25, 29, 92, 109,
    255, 258, 271
Cold War, 141, 159, 190
cortisone, 214, 224–25
Creutzfeldt-Jakob disease, 239
Cushing, Harvey, 103, 106, 111, 225, 227,
    255, 262
Cushing syndrome, 225
Czechoslovakian chickens, 62, 194

D

Daniels, Caroline Seymour, 22
Dartmouth College, 99
Denmark, 147, 245
Desai, Dr. Sukumar, 252
dialysis
    feared, 151

About the Author

SHELLEY FRASER MICKLE is an award-winning novelist whose first novel, *The Queen of October*, was a *New York Times* Notable Book and selected by *Library Journal* as one of the ten best adult books suitable for young adults. Her novel *Replacing Dad* won an America's Writers Award in Chicago and was adapted for film, starring Academy-award nominee Mary McDonnell, airing in March, 1999, on CBS, and re-running on the Hallmark Channel.

The Turning Hour, her novel about a teen suicide attempt based on a true story, was taught in Alachua County Florida schools and was recognized as one of the best tools for suicide prevention in an educational setting by the Florida governor in 2006. Her historical novel set in the Civil War, *The Occupation of Eliza Goode*, was a *Publishers Weekly* and *Huffington Post* Pick of the Week in November, 2013. Her nonfiction book for middle-grade readers, *Barbaro, America's Horse*, won a Bank Street Award, and another middle-grade book, *American Pharaoh, Triple Crown Champion*, was chosen by the New York Public Library as one of the best nonfiction books for children in 2017. From 2000 to 2006 she was a commentator for National Public Radio's *Morning Edition*.

She lives in Gainesville, Florida, and is the mother of two grown children. Her husband trained under the Brigham surgeons who are the focus of this book and retired as a pediatric neurosurgeon from the University of Florida in 2000.